The Best of CRITICAL CARE NURSING

Editor-In-Chief

Cathie E. Guzzetta, RN, PhD, FAAN
Director, Holistic Nursing Consultants, Dallas, Texas

Editors

Tom Ahrens, RN, DNS, CCRN
Clinical Specialist, Critical Care, Barnes Hospital, St. Louis, Missouri

Dorrie Fontaine, RN, DNSc, CCRN
Assistant Professor, Trauma/Critical Care Nursing, University of Maryland, School of Nursing, Baltimore, Maryland

Christine Kessler, RN, MN, CCRN, CS
Manager for Clinical Research, INOVA Health Care Systems, Institute of Research and Education, Falls Church, Virginia; Lecturer, Graduate Faculty, The Catholic University of America, Washington, D.C.

Larry E. Lancaster, RN, MSN, EdD
Associate Professor, Vanderbilt University, School of Nursing, Nashville, Tennessee

Susan F. Wilson, RN, PhD
Associate Professor, Texas Christian University, Harris College of Nursing, Forth Worth, Texas

Sue Wingate, RN, DNSc CCRN, CS
Cardiology Clinical Nurse Specialist, National Institutes of Health, Bethesda, Maryland

Mosby

St. Louis Baltimore Boston Chicago London Philadelphia Sydney Toronto

Editor-in-Chief, Year Book Publishing: Kenneth H. Killion
Sponsoring Editor: Nancy G. Puckett
Manager, Literature Services: Edith M. Podrazik
Senior Information Specialist: Terri Santo
Senior Medical Writer: David A. Cramer, M.D.
Assistant Director, Manuscript Services: Frances M. Perveiler
Associate Managing Editor, Year Book Editing Services: Connie Murray
Senior Production Assistant: Sandra Rogers
Proofroom Manager: Barbara M. Kelly

Mosby
11830 Westline Industrial Drive
St. Louis, MO 63146

Editorial Office:
Mosby
200 North LaSalle St.
Chicago, IL 60601

International Standard Book Number: 0-8151-4014-2

THE BEST OF CRITICAL CARE NURSING

Table of Contents

Journals Regularly Received

Mosby–Year Book subscribes to and surveys nearly 900 U.S. and foreign medical and allied health journals. From these journals, the Editors select the articles to be abstracted.

Acta Cardiologica
Acta Endocrinologica
Acta Neurochirurgica
Acta Neurologica Scandinavica
Acta Obstetricia et Gynecologica Scandinavica
Acta Orthopaedica Scandinavica
Acta Psychiatrica Scandinavica
Acta Radiologica
Advances in Nursing Science
Age-Journal of American Aging Association
Aging, Immunology & Infectious Disease
Age and Aging
Alcohol and Alcoholism
American Family Physician
American Heart Journal
American Industrial Hygiene Association Journal
American Journal of Cardiac Imaging
American Journal of Cardiology
American Journal of Clinical Nutrition
American Journal of Clinical Pathology
American Journal of Critical Care Nursing
American Journal of Emergency Medicine
American Journal of Epidemiology
American Journal of Gastroenterology
American Journal of Hematology
American Journal of Hypertension
American Journal of Infection Control
American Journal of Industrial Medicine
American Journal of Kidney Diseases
American Journal of the Medical Sciences
American Journal of Medicine
American Journal of Medical Sciences
American Journal of Nephrology
American Journal of Neurology
American Journal of Neuroradiology
American Journal of Nursing
American Journal of Obstetrics and Gynecology
American Journal of Occupational Therapy
American Journal of Pediatric Hematology/Oncology
American Journal of Physical Medicine & Rehabilitation
American Journal of Physiology
American Journal of Preventive Medicine
American Journal of Psychiatry
American Journal of Public Health
American Journal of Roentgenology
American Journal of Sports Medicine
American Journal of Surgery
AORN
American Review of Respiratory Disease
American Society of Artificial Internal Organs
American Surgeon

Anaesthesia and Intensive Care
Anesthesia and Analgesia
Anesthesiology
Angiology
Annales Chirurgiae et Gynaecologiae
Annals of Allergy
Annals of Clinical Biochemistry
Annals of Emergency Medicine
Annals of Epidemiology
Annals of Internal Medicine
Annals of Neurology
Annals of Plastic Surgery
Annals of the Royal College of Surgeons of England
Annals of Surgery
Annals of Thoracic Surgery
Annals of Vascular Surgery
Archives of Disease in Childhood
Archives of Emergency Medicine
Archives of General Psychiatry
Archives of Internal Medicine
Archives of Neurology
Archives of Otolaryngology–Head & Neck Surgery
Archives of Pathology and Laboratory Medicine
Archives of Physical Medicine and Rehabilitation
Archives of Surgery
Arteriosclerosis
Arthritis and Rheumatism
Artificial Organs
ASAIO Transactions
Atherosclerosis
Australian and New Zealand Journal of Medicine
Australian and New Zealand Journal of Psychiatry
Behavior Research and Therapy
Biological Psychiatry
Blood
Brain and Cognition
British Heart Journal
British Journal of Cancer
British Journal of Dermatology
British Journal of Genetic Practice
British Journal of Haematology
British Journal of Medical Psychology
British Journal of Plastic Surgery
British Journal of Psychiatry
British Journal of Radiology
British Journal of Surgery
British Journal of Urology
British Medical Journal
Burns
Canadian Association of Radiology Journal
Canadian Family Physician
Canadian Journal of Cardiology
Canadian Journal of Public Health
Canadian Journal of Surgery
Canadian Medical Association Journal

Cancer
Cardiology
Cardiovascular and Interventional Radiology
Cardiovascular Nursing
Cardiovascular Research
Catheterization and Cardiovascular Diagnosis
Chest
Chinese Medical Journal
Chronobiology International
Circulation
Circulation Research
Circulation Supplement
Circulatory Shock
Clinical Chemistry
Clinical Endocrinology
Clinical and Experimental Immunology
Clinical and Experimental Optometry
Clinical Infectious Diseases
Clinical Issues in Critical Care Nursing
Clinical Nephrology
Clinical Nurse Specialist
Clinical Orthopaedics & Related Research
Clinical Otolaryngology
Clinical Pharmacology and Therapeutics
Clinical Physiology
Clinical Science
Complications in Surgery
Contemporary Dialysis and Nephrology
Critical Care Medicine
Critical Care Nurse
Critical Care Nursing Quarterly
Cronobiology International
Cutis
Deutsche Medizinische Wochenschrift
Diabete & Metabolisme
Diabetes Care
Diabetic Medicine
Diabetologia
Diagnostic Microbiology and Infectious Disease
Dialysis and Transplantation
Digestive Diseases and Sciences
Dimensions in Critical Care Nursing
Diseases of the Colon and Rectum
Drug and Alcohol Dependence
Dysphagia
Endocrinology
Epilepsia
European Heart Journal
European Journal of Cancer & Clinical Oncology
European Journal of Clinical Investigation
European Journal of Clinical Pharmacology
European Journal of Haematology
European Journal of Obstetrics, Gynecology & Reproductive Biology
European Journal of Surgery
European Journal of Vascular Surgery

European Respiratory Journal
Family and Community Health Nursing
Family Practice Research Journal
Family Practice
Focus on Critical Care
Gastroenterology
Gastrointestinal Radiology
General Hospital Psychiatry
Genitourinary Medicine
Geriatrics
Geriatric Nurse
Gerontologist
Gut
Headache
Health Care Strategic Management
Health Services Research
Heart Disease and Stroke
Heart and Lung
Hepatology
Holistic Nursing Practice
Hospital and Community Psychiatry
Hospital and Health Services Administration
Human Pathology
Human and Experimental Toxicology
Hypertension
Image
Infection Control
Injury
Inquiry: The Journal of Health Care Organization, Provision, and Financing
Intensive Care Medicine
International Angiology
International Journal of Artificial Organs
International Journal of Cardiology
International Journal of Eating Disorders
International Journal of Epidemiology
International Journal of Gynecological Pathology
International Journal of Health Services
International Journal of Nursing Studies
International Journal of Pancreatology
Investigative Radiology
Israel Journal of Medical Sciences
Italian Journal of Neurological Sciences
Journal of Acquired Immune Deficiency Syndromes
Journal of Advanced Nursing
Journal of Allergy & Clinical Immunology
Journal of the American Academy of Physician Assistance
Journal of the American College of Cardiology
Journal of the American Geriatrics Society
Journal of the American Medical Association
Journal of the American Nephrology Nurses (ANNA)
Journal of the American Osteopathic Association
Journal of the American Society of Nephrology
Journal of Antimicrobial Chemotherapy
Journal of Applied Behavioral Analysis
Journal of Applied Physiology

Journal of Arthroplasty
Journal of Bone and Joint Surgery (American vol.)
Journal of Bone and Joint Surgery (British vol.)
Journal of Burn Care Rehabilitation
Journal of Cardiac Surgery
Journal of Cardiopulmonary Rehabilitation
Journal of Cardiovascular Nursing
Journal of Cardiovascular Surgery
Journal de Chirurgie
Journal of Clinical Endocrinology & Metabolism
Journal of Enterostomal Therapy Nursing
Journal of Clinical Epidemiology
Journal of Clinical Gastroenterology
Journal of Clinical Immunology
Journal of Obstetrics/Gynecology Nursing (JOGNN)
Journal of Clinical Pathology
Journal of Clinical Pharmacology
Journal of Clinical Pharmacy and Therapeutics
Journal of Clinical Psychiatry
Journal of Clinical Research and Pharmacoepidemiology
Journal of Clinical Ultrasound
Journal of Consulting and Clinical Psychology
Journal of Dermatology
Journal of Electrocardiology
Journal of Emergency Medicine
Journal of Emergency Nursing
Journal of Family Practice
Journal of Gerontology
Journal of Health and Social Behavior
Journal of Heart and Lung Transplantation
Journal of Human Hypertension
Journal of Infectious Diseases
Journal of Intensive Care Medicine
Journal of Internal Medicine
Journal of Interventional Cardiology
Journal of Intravenous Nursing
Journal of Laryngology and Otology
Journal of the National Cancer Institute
Journal of Neurological Sciences
Journal of Neurological Surgical Nursing
Journal of Neurology, Neurosurgery and Psychiatry
Journal of Neuroscience Nursing
Journal of Neurosurgery
Journal of Nuclear Medicine
Journal of Nursing Administration
Journal of Nursing Education
Journal of Nursing Quality Assurance
Journal of Oral and Maxillofacial Surgery
Journal of Orthopaedic Trauma
Journal of Pain and Symptom Management
Journal of Pediatric Health Care
Journal of Physical Medicine Rehabilitation
Journal of Post-Anesthetic Nursing
Journal of Professional Nursing
Journal of Psychiatric Medical Rehabilitation

Journal of Psychological Nursing and Mental Health Services
Journal of Rehabilitation
Journal of Reproductive Medicine
Journal of Rheumatology
Journal of the Royal College of Surgeons of Edinburgh
Journal of the Royal Society of Medicine
Journal of Speech and Hearing Research
Journal of Surgical Research
Journal of Thoracic and Cardiovascular Surgery
Journal of Trauma
Journal of Urology
Journal of Vascular Surgery
Kidney International
Klinische Wochenschrift
Lancet
Laryngoscope
Law, Medicine and Health Care
Liver
LaPrisse Medicule
Magnetic Resonance Imaging
Mayo Clinic Proceedings
Medical Care
Medical Journal of Australia
Medicine
Medicine and Science in Sports and Exercise
Metabolism
Mineral and Electrolyte Metabolism
Mount Sinai Journal of Medicine (New York)
Muscle & Nerve
Nephrology Dialysis Transplantation
Nephron
Neurochirurgia
Neurology
Neuroradiology
Neurosurgery
New England Journal of Medicine
New England Journal of Optometry
New York State Journal of Medicine
Nuclear Medicine
Nursing '91
Nursing Clinics of North America
Nursing Diagnosis
Nursing and Health Care
Nursing Management
Nursing Outlook
Nursing Research
Obstetrics and Gynecology
Oncology Nursing Forum
Opthalmology
Orthopaedic Review
Pace
Pacing and Clinical Electrophysiology
Pain
Paraplegia
Patient Education and Counseling

Pediatric Infectious Disease
Pediatric Neurology
Pharmacotherapy
Physician and Sportsmedicine
Postgraduate Medical Journal
Postgraduate Medicine
Progress in Cardiovascular Nursing
Prosthetics and Orthotics International
Psychological Assessment
Psychosomatic Medicine
Public Health Reports
Quarterly Journal of Medicine
Radiology
Research in Nursing and in Health
Respiratory Medicine
Reviews of Infectious Diseases
RN
S.A.M.J./S.A.M.T.–South African Medical Journal
Scandinavian Journal of Clinical Laboratory Investigation
Scandinavian Journal of Gastroenterology
Scandinavian Journal of Infectious Disease
Scandinavian Journal of Primary Health Care
Scandinavian Journal of Rehabilitation Medicine
Scandinavian Journal of Thoracic and Cardiovascular Surgery
Scandinavian Journal of Urology and Nephrology
Scandinavian Journal of Work Environment and Health
Scholarly Inquiry for Nursing Practice
Schweizerische Medizinische Wochenschrift
Science
Semaine des Hopitaux
Semaine des Hopitaux Paris
Sourth African Medical Journal
Southern Medical Journal
Spine
Sports Medicine
Sports Training, Medicine, and Rehabilitation
Stroke
Surgery
Surgery, Gynecology and Obstetrics
Surgical Neurology
Surgical Research Communications
Therapeutic Drug Monitoring
Thorax
Thrombosis and Haemostasis
Transactions of the AMSAID (Am. Soc. for Artificial Internal Organs)
Transfusion
Transplantation
Transplantation Proceedings
Tubercle
Trauma Quarterly
Urology
Vascular Surgery
Virchows Archiv A: Pathological Anatomy and Histopathology
Vox Sanguinis
Western Journal of Medicine

Western Journal of Nursing Research
Wiener Klinische Wochenschrift
Yale Journal of Biology and Medicine

STANDARD ABBREVIATIONS

The following terms are abbreviated in this edition: acquired immunodeficiency syndrome (AIDS), the central nervous system (CNS), cerebrospinal fluid (CSF), computed tomography (CT), electrocardiography (ECG), human immunodeficiency virus (HIV), and magnetic resonance (MR) imaging (MRI).

AACN Research Priorities

Priority areas for critical care nursing research were identified at a recently completed Research Priorities Consensus Conference in Orlando, Florida.

Sponsored by the American Association of Critical Care Nurses (AACN) and held in conjunction with its annual Leadership Institute, a panel of 50 critical care nurse experts from across the nation determined the priority listings.

Research topics were identified and prioritized in two categories—clinical practice and the context within which critical care nursing takes place.

Priorities for clinical practice research in critical care nursing are:

- Techniques to optimize pulmonary functioning and prevent pulmonary complications
- Weaning of mechanically ventilated patients
- Effect of nursing activities/interventions on hemodynamic parameters
- Techniques for real-time monitoring of tissue perfusion and oxygenation
- Nutritional support modalities and patient outcomes
- Interventions to prevent infection
- Pain assessment and pain management techniques
- Accuracy and precision of invasive and non-invasive monitoring devices
- Effect of nursing activities, environmental stimuli and human interactions on intracranial and cerebral perfusion pressure

Priorities for research on the context within which critical care nursing takes place are:

- Incorporation of research findings into critical care nursing practice
- Levels of nursing competence (e.g., certification) and the effect on patient outcomes
- Occupational hazards (e.g., HIV, noise, substance abuse, premature delivery)
- Ethical issues related to initiation, maintenance and withdrawal of life support technology (e.g., living wills)
- Patient care delivery models for critical care
- Collaboration and communication among health care professionals
- Role of critical care nurses in decisions regarding resuscitation status of critically ill patients

Before the conference, prior and current critical care research was summarized to identify areas where research is needed. In a nationwide survey, critical care nurses rated the perceived importance of each possible research area. Using the survey data, the AACN Research Committee developed the topic lists that were prioritized at the conference.

Dedication

This book is dedicated to our critical care nursing colleagues and their patients.

Acknowledgments

We are indebted to Mosby's Year Book team who had the vision and then gave us the latitude to transform the traditional flagship medical publication into a nursing reality.

For their assistance, guidance, and direction in this project, we thank Nancy Gorham, Nancy Puckett, Edie Podrazik, Ken Killion, and Deirdre Bryan.

We thank each of the families of the Editors of Mosby's BEST OF CRITICAL CARE NURSING for their patience, support, and understanding in seeing us through just one more project.

Introduction

Can you imagine surveying 400 journals in a year? Well, that's what we did. In preparation for this YEAR BOOK, Mosby headquarters sent me critical care articles that were published in 400 American and foreign nursing, health care management, and medical journals over the past year. I received shipments of articles every other week and then triaged specific articles to the other 6 Editors. In a 1-year period, I had received approximately 6,500 articles, which when placed in a single stack, reached a height of 8½ feet!

Our job then was to plow through and critically review these articles, eliminate 98.5% of them, and select the top 100 articles from this stack to share with you. The articles were professionally abstracted to provide you with a skillful distillation that preseves the content of the article and yet allows you to get the meat of the information in only a few minutes. In addition, we wrote commentaries on how this information is significant in day-to-day critical care nursing practice. Our focus was to provide relevance, insight, clarification, and alternative perspectives in clinical practice. For example, how might this information change what we do at the bedside? And why is it significant? When commenting on a medical article, we explored why this information is important to nurses (i.e., how can this *medical* information be viewed from a *nursing perspective* and what are the implications for nursing practice). Moreover, we also directed our comments to the strengths and weaknesses of the article, frequently giving you our vision of what might work or what problems still exist in the area. That is what this book is all about.

The YEAR BOOK concept may be new to some of you. YEAR BOOKS have been popular in medicine and surgery for nearly 100 years. The first YEAR BOOK (on nose, throat, and ear) was published in 1901 and was developed to be the "epitome of the best literature of the year put into a volume convenient for reference." Currently there are 45 annual YEAR BOOKS in various medical and surgical specialties read worldwide and translated into a number of foreign languages. This volume, however, represents the first YEAR BOOK written for nurses by nurses.

Why might this YEAR BOOK be important to you? The literature in critical care nursing and medicine is exploding. There is tremendous pressure for all nurses to keep up with the latest advances in their field (e.g., for reasons of accountability, evaluation, promotion, certification, and accreditation). It is impossible to stay on top of the latest trends, newest advances, and current developments in the ever-changing world of critical care when there are thousands of critical care articles published in hundreds of journals each year. The 7 of us were brought together to do this job because it is virtually impossible for any *one person* to keep up-to-date with this overflow of literature.

This book focuses on adult critically ill patients and their nurse caregivers. It is intended for all students, practitioners, educators, and researchers who are interested in updating and expanding their critical care knowledge. We have used an enormously large literature base to provide an overview of clinically applicable advances in critical care nursing. The abstracted articles reflect physiologic and psychosocial patient care problems as well as current caregiver issues related to critical care practice (e.g., research, quality assurance, safety, standards, educational, role, administrative, financial, technological, and environmental issues). Useful figures, tables, grafts, and charts also are included. A unique strength of this project is the clinical diversity of the Editorial Board — each of whom is nationally recognized as an expert in critical care nursing.

Because we found the critical care literature to be even more voluminous than we imagined, we have decided to continue this work via a quarterly journal format. Thus, current articles and commentaries will reach you even faster in our new CAPSULES AND COMMENTS IN CRITICAL CARE NURSING, which also premieres this month.

The information age of the 90s is upon us. The boundaries by which the critical care literature will expand in the future remain limitless. It is our hope that we can assist you in managing the knowledge explosion. We also hope that some of the articles and commentaries in this book and in CAPSULES AND COMMENTS IN CRITICAL CARE NURSING will update you and, perhaps even inspire you, to provide better quality patient care.

Cathie E. Guzzetta
Editor-in-Chief

PATIENT PROBLEMS

1 Cardiovascular Dysfunction

Hemodynamic Monitoring

Comparison of Thermodilution and Transthoracic Electrical Bioimpedance Cardiac Outputs

Woo MA, Hamilton M, Stevenson LW, Vredevoe DL (Univ of California, Los Angeles)

Heart Lung 20:357–362, 1991 1–1

Problem.—The thermodilution (TD) catheter is the most commonly used tool for measuring cardiac output in critically ill patients; however, this technique is invasive and carries serious risks. One suggested alternative is transthoracic electric bioimpedance (TEB), a noninvasive tool. These 2 measurement techniques were compared in patients in a coronary care unit.

Methods.—The 44 patients, selected for convenience, all had poor left ventricular function and ischemic or idiopathic dilated cardiomyopathy.

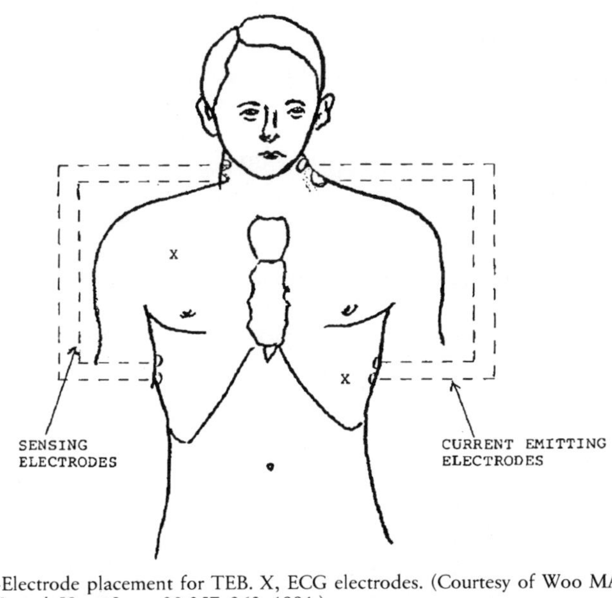

Fig 1–1.—Electrode placement for TEB. X, ECG electrodes. (Courtesy of Woo MA, Hamilton M, Stevenson LW, et al: *Heart Lung* 20:357–362, 1991.)

For each patient, cardiac output measurement by TEB was performed within 1 minute after each TD injection. Reliability of both methods was established; sensitivity of the TEB device was ensured by correct placement of the electrodes (Fig 1–1). A total of 80 readings—2 sets of readings in 36 patients and 1 set in 8 patients—were included in the final analysis. Twenty-three variables previously identified as possible threats to the validity of TEB were analyzed for their effects on the correlation between the methods.

Findings.—More than two thirds of TEB readings were more than .5 L/min different from the simultaneous TD cardiac outputs. The 2 methods were significantly correlated, but not at a level high enough for clinical significance. In addition, TEB had a low reliability. The correlation between the 2 methods was most affected by dyspnea, mitral regurgitation, tricuspid regurgitation, and the difference between real and ideal weight. Left ventricular ejection fraction, height, weight, hemoglobin, hematocrit, and aortic regurgitation had lesser effects on the correlation.

Conclusions.—Transthoracic electric bioimpedance is insufficient compared to TD for clinical measurement of cardiac output in critically ill patients. This is especially true for taller, heavier patients with dyspnea and significant mitral or tricuspid valve regurgitation. When TEB is used, the nurse should be careful to document the patient's condition from more viewpoints than just skin impedance.

Comments: Despite the lack of a clinically significant correlation between the TEB and TD methods of cardiac output measurement, this study has great importance for critical care nurses. The technology of TEB must be investigated because it is the wave of the future—pulmonary artery catheters will not be around forever. To be able to obtain similar parameters with noninvasive monitoring as those obtained with invasive monitoring will drastically alter patient management in the future. As with other technology, TEB is in the early stages of development and use and so, *now is the time for nurses and other users to critically evaluate it*—otherwise it will enter our practice setting without our input.

Other studies have looked at TEB and similar noninvasive measures of hemodynamic parameters. Accurate systolic and diastolic time intervals by TEB (1) and clinically significant correlations in cardiac output by TEB (2) have been found in critically ill patients. Doppler ultrasound with aortic blood flow velocity and waveform variables has been found to provide accurate measurements of left ventricular preload, afterload, and contractility in healthy subjects (3). In addition, TEB has been found to cost $600 less than TD methods (2).

These authors are to be commended for studying the technology of TEB in a different population. New technology often makes its way into the clinical arena after being tested on only some sectors of the population and then is assumed to be reliable for all patients. This area should be one of nursing's primary clinical research efforts—validating the use of potentially beneficial technology with different patient populations and assessing its effects on patient outcomes, cost, time, and nursing education. In fact, this area was listed as one of the priorities for critical care nursing research by the American Association of Critical-Care Nurses (4). If noninvasive measurements of hemodynamics become more accurate and reliable in various critical care patient populations, it will be a boon for both patients and nurses. Less cost and risk to the patient. Less time for nurses. It's worth studying.—S. Wingate, RN, DNSc, CCRN, CS

References

1. Mattar JO, Shoemaker WC, Diament D, et al: Systolic and diastolic time intervals in the critically ill patient. *Crit Care Med* 19:1382, 1991.
2. Clancy TV, Norman K, Reynolds R, et al: Cardiac output measurement in critical care patients: Thoracic electrical bioimpedance versus thermodilution. *J Trauma* 31:1116, 1991.
3. Singer M, Allen MJ, Webb AR, et al: Effects of alterations in left ventricular filling, contractility, and systemic vascular resistance on the ascending aortic blood velocity waveform of normal subjects. *Crit Care Med* 19:1138, 1991.
4. Press Release, American Association of Critical-Care Nurses, Aliso Viejo, CA, November 21, 1991.

Current Practice Regarding Invasive Monitoring in Intensive Care Units in Finland: A Nationwide Study of the Uses of Arterial, Pulmonary Artery and Central Venous Catheters and Their Effect on Outcome

Saarela E, for the Finnish Intensive Care Study Group (Oulu Univ, Oulu, Finland)

Intensive Care Med 17:264–271, 1991 1–2

Problem.—Invasive monitoring techniques such as pulmonary artery (PA) catheters are widely used in critical care, even when their clinical effectiveness has not been proved in randomized studies. Factors influencing the use of these techniques and their effect on outcome in critically ill patients were investigated.

Study Methods.—The study, which was part of a nationwide evaluation of intensive care, included 13,400 patients admitted to 25 intensive care units (ICUs). Burn and postoperative cardiac patients were excluded. The use of arterial cannulas and central venous pressure (CVP) and PA catheters at each center was assessed. Factors associated with different patterns of use were also analyzed. Logistic multiple regression analysis was done to assess the effect of these monitoring techniques on patient outcome.

Findings.—In teaching ICUs, approximately 71% used arterial cannulation, 10% used PA catheterization, and 50% used CVP monitoring. In nonteaching ICUs, the approximate figures were 39%, 3%, and 33%, respectively. Invasive monitoring was unrelated to effectiveness of care; that is, hospital mortality rates were unchanged. Arterial cannulas were most often used in postoperative patients; in nonoperative patients, arterial cannulas were generally used only for respiratory failure caused by infection or pancreatitis. Pulmonary artery catheters were usually used for nonoperative patients, except for neurosurgery. Central venous pressure monitoring was most often done in patients with sepsis, emergency abdominal surgery, and pancreatitis.

Conclusions.—The use of invasive monitoring appears to be based mainly on clinical needs, but also on tradition. Such monitoring does not appear to improve the short-term outcome of decreased hospital mortality rates or to increase the intensity of therapy. Invasive monitoring is most popular in the care of postoperative patients in teaching ICUs.

Comments: Hemodynamic monitoring with invasive catheters is a major component of an ICU nurse's job. For something that consumes so much of our time, one would hope that it produces worthwhile benefits to the patient. Saarela et al. provide interesting food for thought in this area. First, they found that placement of invasive monitoring devices had no effect on hospital mortality. Granted, this study was done in Finland, and it was also done in 1986 and 1987—2 factors that limit the study's generalizability to present day care in the United States. However, I think their results are dramatic enough for us to think about seriously.

If such invasive procedures do not decrease hospital mortality, then one wonders whether their cost and risks are truly justified. Further, although it is recognized that invasive monitoring itself is not a therapeutic measure, it should *lead* to therapeutic interventions. However, these investigators found no difference in the intensity of treatment given to patients whether or not they received invasive monitoring.

A second interesting finding was that invasive monitoring was used more often in postoperative patients in teaching hospitals than in nonteaching hospitals, despite there being a higher proportion of seriously ill patients in nonteaching ICUs. So. . . do teaching ICUs do too much or do nonteaching ICUs do too little? This is an interesting question considering there was no difference in mortality between the 2 settings.

It is recognized that other studies have shown a significant impact on treatment with invasive monitoring (1,2). With such conflicting findings, however, the clinician is left wondering what to believe. Further, mortality may not be the only outcome to study. Perhaps interventions resulting from invasive monitoring improved symptoms, decreased morbidity, or enhanced quality of life. This is not known from the present study.

As critical care nurses, we serve as advocates for the patient and family. We must keep abreast of these research findings to best guide patients in their decision-making. Is the technology really worth the discomfort, cost, and possible risks? Does it really have an impact on patient outcomes—both quantitative and qualitative? Should you see more invasive monitoring just because you work in a teaching ICU? As these authors stated, it may be time for a randomized trial of invasive monitoring to assess its true benefits. As nurses, although we can't prescribe medical treatment, we can certainly study the outcome of patients who were or who were not monitored invasively. We have to—we can't let technology get ahead of us.—S. Wingate, RN, DNSc, CCRN, CS

References

1. Eisenberg PR, Jaffe AS, Schuster DP: Clinical evaluation compared to pulmonary artery catheterization in the hemodynamic assessment of critically ill patients. *Crit Care Med* 12:549, 1984.
2. Tuchschmidt J, Sharma OP: Impact of hemodynamic monitoring in a medical intensive care unit. *Crit Care Med* 15:840, 1987.

Interobserver Variability in the Interpretation of Pulmonary Artery Catheter Pressure Tracings

Komadina KH, Schenk DA, LaVeau P, Duncan CA, Chambers SL (Wilford Hall USAF Med Ctr; Univ of Texas, San Antonio; Audie Murphy VA Hosp, San Antonio)

Chest 100:1647–1654, 1991 1–3

Problem.—Much information on hemodynamic parameters is gained by the use of pulmonary artery (PA) catheters in the medical and surgical intensive care units (ICU). However, studies have failed to demonstrate any consistent improvement in survival among patients managed with a

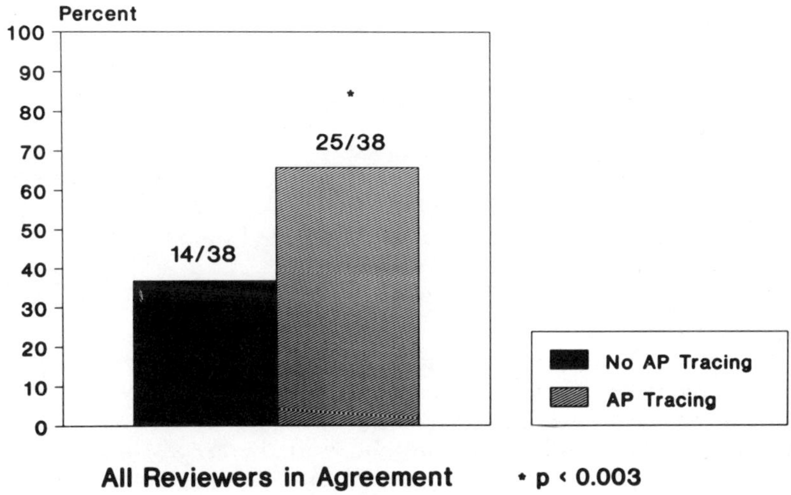

Fig 1–2.—Agreement (%) by all 3 reviewers in assessing the validity of the PCWP tracings using waveform analysis is shown. Only confirmed-valid tracings were analyzed (n = 38). All 3 reviewers correctly identified 14 of 38 (37%) confirmed-valid tracings when analyzed without an AP tracing to define end-expiration. Agreement by all 3 reviewers was significantly increased when the same tracings were reviewed with an AP tracing. Twenty-five of 38 (66%) confirmed-valid tracings were correctly identified in this setting ($P < .003$). (Courtesy of Komadina KH, Schenk DA, LaVeau P, et al: *Chest* 100:1647–1654, 1991.)

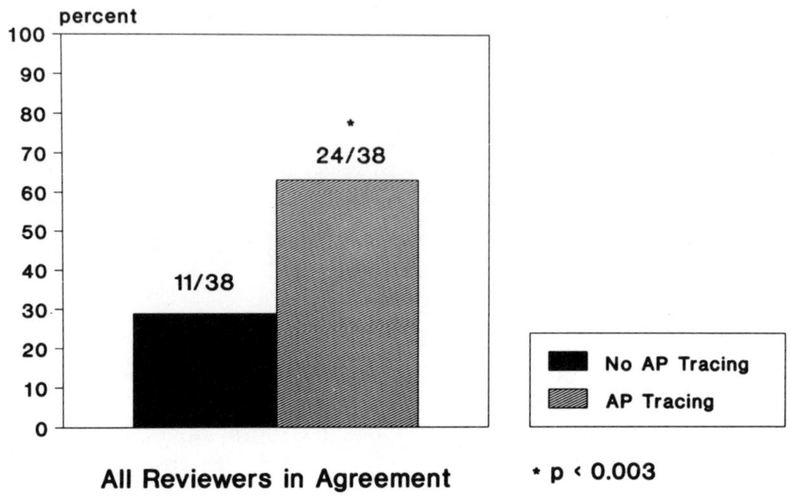

Fig 1–3.—Agreement (%) by all 3 reviewers on the PCWP numerical reading is shown. Only confirmed-valid tracings were analyzed (n = 38). Without the use of an AP tracing to define end-expiration, agreement was achieved in 11 of 38 (29%) confirmed-valid tracings. With the use of an AP tracing, all 3 reviewers agreed in 24 of 38 (63%) confirmed-valid tracings ($P < .003$). (Courtesy of Komadina KH, Schenk DA, LaVeau P, et al: *Chest* 100:1647–1654, 1991.)

PA catheter. A study was done to determine whether independent reviewers could accurately identify confirmed valid pulmonary capillary wedge pressure (PCWP) tracings and whether they were consistently able to report the numerical value of the PCWP.

Study Methods.—Data were gathered on 20 patients with 22 PA catheters. All patients were undergoing mechanical ventilation. Rigorous techniques were used to obtain the PA catheter measurements and to validate the position of the PA catheter with aspiration of pulmonary capillary blood. A total of 60 tracings were obtained and reviewed in blinded fashion by 3 critical care physicians—2 pulmonologists and 1 cardiologist. Thirty-eight tracings were confirmed valid by blood analysis, and 22 were unconfirmed. The physicians reviewed each tracing, first without an airway pressure (AP) tracing and then again with an AP tracing.

Findings.—Thirty-seven percent of confirmed valid tracings were identified correctly by all 3 reviewers using waveform analysis. When the same tracings were reviewed with an AP tracing to define end-expiration, 66% of confirmed valid tracings were identified correctly by all 3 reviewers (Fig 1–2). Reviewer accuracy for waveform analysis ranged from 50% to 65%. The 3 reviewers agreed on the numerical PCWP in 29% of the confirmed valid tracings. When the same tracings were reviewed with an AP tracing, the reviewers agreed on 63% of the tracings (Fig 1–3). However, of the confirmed valid tracings that the reviewers noted as valid by waveform analysis, they agreed on the numerical PCWP reading in 79%

of the tracings without AP analysis and 96% of the tracings with AP analysis. The numerical readings of ICU nurses and house officers correlated closely with the reviewer's readings.

Conclusion.—Proper and consistent interpretation of PA catheter tracings is vital to therapeutic decision-making; however, physician reviewer waveform analysis to predict confirmed valid tracings is subjective and is a little better than a random guess. Pressure data obtained by a PA catheter should be viewed in the context of all clinical data and should not be relied on as the sole measure of a patient's status.

Comments: It's scary to think that therapeutic decisions are made according to data that may be no better than a random guess. Despite the fact that this investigation's data represent measurements on only 20 patients, the rigorous design of the study strengthens the findings. It is recognized that this study did not evaluate decision-making or mortality, but one is inclined to try to connect these 2 issues. Are inaccurate readings somehow tied to wrong therapeutic decisions that then fail to improve patient survival? This is a big leap but not totally unjustified, considering reports that invasive monitoring may not improve patient mortality (see Abstract 1–2). The authors may indeed be correct in calling for a randomized trial on the efficacy of pulmonary artery catheters. What also is needed, however, is some evaluation of how pressure data are integrated with other patient assessment data for clinical decision-making.

Even though this study was concerned with physicians, the nursing implications are obvious. Although not detailed, the study noted that ICU nurses' readings were similar to those of the critical care physicians, and thus had a poor accuracy rate. Why is this? Are we not rigorous enough in our measurements? Were we taught in the correct way, both didactically and at the bedside? Do we integrate pressure data with other assessment data or do we put too much faith in technology alone?

This study should be replicated in other settings using other equipment to validate the findings. This is a study *begging* to be done by critical care nurses—it is our territory.—S. Wingate, RN, DNSc, CCRN, CS

A Meta-Analysis of Effects of Heparin Flush and Saline Flush: Quality and Cost Implications

Goode CJ, Titler M, Rakel B, Ones DS, Kleiber C, Small S, Triolo PK (Univ of Iowa Hosps and Clinics)

Nurs Res 40:324–330, 1991 1–4

Problem.—Because controversy continues over which type of irrigating solution to use with heparin locks, data were reviewed from 17 studies that used an experimental or quasi-experimental design to estimate the effects of heparin- and saline-flush solutions on patency, the occurrence of phlebitis, and the duration of peripheral heparin locks.

Annual Cost Savings From Changing to Saline

Study	Cost Savings	Hospital
Craig & Anderson, 1991	$40,000/yr	525-bed tertiary care hospital
Dunn & Lenihan, 1987	$19,000/yr	530-bed private hospital
Goode et al., 1991 (this study)	$38,000/yr	879-bed tertiary care hospital
Kasparek et al., 1988	$19,000/yr	350- bed private hospital
Lombardi et al., 1988	$20,000–$25,000/yr	52-bed pediatric unit
Schustek, 1984	$20,000/yr	391-bed private hospital
Taylor et al., 1989	$30,000–$40,000/yr	216-bed private hospital

(Courtesy of Goode CJ, Titler M, Rakel B, et al: *Nurs Res* 40:324–330, 1991.)

Study Methods.—The 17 studies were reviewed using meta-analysis techniques. Each study was classified according to sample size, type of subjects, site of study, and dosage of heparin.

Findings.—There was no conclusive evidence that heparin prevents clotting more effectively than saline, or that it is better in preventing phlebitis. Saline was as effective as heparin in lengthening the duration of a lock. There were substantial cost savings in using a saline flush including supplies, drugs, and staff time (table). If each acute care hospital in the United States saved from $19,000 to $40,000 annually, nearly $220 million would be saved each year nationwide.

Recommendations for Practice.—A saline-flush solution is preferable to heparin solution for flushing peripheral intravenous locks, although these results should not be extended to children or neonates. Further studies are needed to determine how frequently locks should be irrigated with saline.

Comments: Why are practice patterns different from hospital to hospital? Shouldn't patients expect to receive the same care whether they are in one institution versus another? And why should nurses relearn how to do something when they go to work somewhere else, simply because "that's the way we do it here?" It all relates, I think, to not having a scientific basis for our practice. We do things because we extrapolate from other studies or because "we've always done them that way."

These authors did something that is sorely needed in nursing—a meta-analysis for all the studies on a particular issue to come up with recommendations for practice based on science. That a review of 17 studies showed no benefit of heparin over saline in patency, or duration of peripheral intravenous locks, or the development of phlebitis is remarkable clinical information.

As the authors noted, the cost-savings implications are significant—decreased cost of supplies and drugs as well as nursing time. In addition, there is decreased risk for the patient in terms of preventing potential anticoagulant effects and drug incompatibilities.

Two important issues arise from the findings of this meta-analysis. First, it opens up questions for further research. We still need to know the frequency and amount of saline irrigation that is needed, and we need to explore how these data relate to central infusion devices or to hemodynamic monitoring devices. It is important to note, however, the results of the American Association of Critical Care Nurses' "Thunder Project" on saline versus heparin in arterial lines revealed that heparinized flush solutions increased the chance for patency in arterial catheters (1). A report of the Thunder Project will be published in January 1993 issue of the *American Journal of Critical Care.*

Second, what is the best way to disseminate this information? Information certainly needs to get to the bedside clinicians and nursing leadership in hospitals where heparin is used as a peripheral flush solution. It also needs to get to the physicians who routinely order the heparin flushes, and they need to know that *nursing research* is what caused the change. This is quite a challenge. Any ideas?—S. Wingate, RN, DNSc, CCRN, CS

Reference

1. American Association of Critical-Care Nurses: Press release, Thunder Project. Aliso Viejo, Calif, November 5, 1992.

Nursing Observations of Central Venous Catheters: The Effect on Patient Outcome

Capka MB, Carey S, Marks D, Wilson M, Benard J (Emory Univ, Atlanta)
J Intravenous Nurs 14:243–246, 1991 1–5

Problem.—Central venous catheters (CVCs), although a routine and valuable part of nursing care, are a major source of infection and septicemia. A descriptive investigation of how nursing management of patients with CVCs affected infection rates on the general nursing units was conducted.

Methods.—Included were 43 adults with nonimplantable catheters in place for longer than 48 hours. Thirteen were admitted for acute medical conditions; 11 each were admitted for oncologic and chronic medical conditions; and 8 for surgical conditions. Using flowsheets during a 6-week period, nursing staff collected data on diagnosis, reason for insertion, risk factors, length of indwelling time, type of dressing, site condition, frequency of dressing and tubing changes, and number of system entries.

Findings.—Data on 52 catheter insertions and 567 line days were analyzed. The most common reasons for CVC insertion were fluid maintenance, medication administration, or both (table). In 26 patients, periph-

Rationale for Central-Line Insertion and Identified Risk Factors Associated With Potential Infection (N = 52)

	n	%
Rationale for Insertion		
Medications/fluids	31	59.6
Inadequate peripheral sites	26	50.0
Hyperalimentation	22	42.3
Blood/blood products	3	5.8
Chemotherapy	2	3.8
Risk Factors Present in the Sample		
Antibiotics	29	55.8
Hyperalimentation	14	26.9
Diabetes	10	19.2
Steroid therapy	5	9.6
Previous site contamination	4	7.7
Chemotherapy	3	5.8
Neutropenia	3	5.8
AIDS	2	3.8
Tracheotomy	2	3.8

(Courtesy of Capka MB, Carey S, Marks D, et al: *J Intravenous Nurs* 14:243–246, 1991.)

eral sites were inadequate. Antibiotic therapy was the most frequent risk factor. Most catheters were inserted by physicians at the bedside or in the operating room. Catheters were in place an average of 10.9 days, and occlusive gauze dressings were used in almost every patient. The average number of needle entries was 180. Seven sites (13.4%) showed redness after 8 days, and all but 2 of the catheters were removed after these signs of site irritation. These 2 cases resulted in catheter-related septicemia; no definitive trends could be identified explaining why these infections occurred.

Conclusions.—In patients with CVCs, careful nursing observation and documentation with aggressive follow-up when signs of impending infection appear may avert systemic infection. When irritation of the insertion site is noted, the catheter should be removed promptly. Policies regarding frequent line changes may need reevaluation in light of the finding that these patients averaged almost 11 days per catheter with infrequent adverse consequences.

Comments: What a great example of a simple, practical clinical nursing research project! These authors chose an important and costly patient outcome—CVC infections—and described how *routine* nursing care affected this outcome. Thus, they took the first step in examining how their practice could be modified to decrease costs while enhancing patient outcomes—very timely in these days of cost containment.

The nursing care outcomes of this study are quite significant. Of the catheters that were noted to have site irritations and were removed, there were no infection-related problems. Despite nursing documentation and communication of site problems with 2 catheters, however, these catheters were not removed and eventually caused septicemia. The reader can only wonder why the communication was not effective in getting the catheter removed. There are also important financial implications of this study. If catheters truly do not need to be changed as frequently as some hospital policies state, resources are conserved (supplies, nursing time) and patient discomfort is alleviated.

This project originated from the Nursing Research Committee, but the data were collected by the staff on the involved units. This not only allowed them to evaluate their practice critically but also gave them some ownership in sharing the study's results and disseminating the findings. This type of staff participation is really the only way that nursing research can be actualized in the clinical setting. The findings of this study certainly should be replicated before broad changes are recommended for nursing practice. However, these authors have taken an important first step in describing their practice and its effects on patient outcomes. They showed that nursing care clearly made a difference. Again, we know how critical the work we do is, but these authors took the time to prove it.—S. Wingate, RN, DNSc, CCRN, CS

Partial Occlusion of Indwelling Central Venous Catheters

Lawson M (Ivion Corp, Englewood, Colo)

J Intravenous Nurs 14:157–159, 1991 1–6

Problem.—The number of central venous catheters (CVCs) used for long-term continuous or long-term intermittent infusions in high-risk patients has increased in the past 10 years. The many problems associated with long-term indwelling CVC use initially prompted removal of the catheter. However, research and experience have shown that these catheters can often be salvaged without endangering the patient.

Methods and Findings.—In 10 patients with an indwelling CVC, the catheters were explanted because blood could not be aspirated from the otherwise patent CVC. Examination of the CVCs indicated no blood clot or fibrin sheath formation at the catheter tip. External defects also were not seen on any CVC or port. Blood product deposits were seen in each of the halved CVCs at the junction of the catheter and catheter hub and in the dead space at the base of each port housing. A second group of 10 patients who had difficulties with catheter aspiration were studied to identify the best intervention for this problem. Normal saline flushes did not prevent or correct the problem. Use of a fibrinolytic drug (urokinase) successfully cleared all CVCs. Use of prophylactic urokinase also maintained catheter patency between monthly usages.

Recommendations.—A fibrinolytic drug with an established declotting procedure should be used to correct the problem of CVCs partially occluded with blood products. Such a drug should also be used prophylactically to cleanse the indwelling CVC periodically of all accumulated blood or blood products. Controlled studies also should be conducted to determine the incidence of partially occluded indwelling CVCs, the incidence of CVC loss because of partial occlusion, and the incidence of associated CVC infections. Studies should also be conducted to determine how frequently the indwelling CVC should be cleaned with a fibrinolytic drug.

Comments: Central venous catheters have become an important part of infusion therapy, especially in high-risk populations, such as critically ill and immunocompromised patients. Many of these patients also have poor venous access and thus use the CVC for blood sampling. When these catheters malfunction, catheter removal and reinsertion can cause patient discomfort, delays in therapy, and increased costs.

This paper reports on studies done in patients with CVCs that showed that deposits of blood products in the CVCs and their implanted ports may act like a ball valve when aspiration is attempted and, thus, prevent aspiration. Possible solutions were discussed, and in a subsequent study, it was found that the use of urokinase, a fibrinolytic drug, successfully cleared all CVCs, enabling blood aspirations. The author recommended use of a fibrinolytic drug for both prophylactic and as-needed use in CVCs.

If replicated in larger, controlled studies, this procedure would greatly improve the care of patients with indwelling CVCs, especially in the critical care area. Patients would be spared the discomfort of interim peripheral venipunctures, therapy would not be interrupted because of catheter malfunction, and cost savings would be realized if catheters did not need replacement.

Many aspects of this problem with CVCs still need investigation: What is the real incidence of the problem? Are there other methods for resolving occluded catheters? What is the cost-benefit analysis? What is the best declotting procedure? Are there any complications or contraindications to declotting CVCs? What is the patient response to problems with their CVCs? What a fruitful area for clinical nursing research!—S. Wingate, RN, DNSc, CCRN, CS

Dysrhythmias

Clinical Decision Making of Critical Care Nurses Managing Computer-Simulated Tachydysrhythmias

Henry SB (Univ of California, San Francisco)
Heart Lung 20:469–477, 1991 1–7

Problem.—Little is known about clinical decision-making by nurses, particularly critical care nurses. The clinical decision-making of critical care nurses in the management of computer-simulated tachydysrhythmias was evaluated and the major sources of errors related to dysrhythmia management were determined.

Study Methods.—The descriptive study included 142 critical care nurses, each of whom completed 4 computerized clinical simulations. There were 2 simulations each of atrial flutter and ventricular tachycardia, chosen to represent different levels of patient acuity. The nurses' performance on these simulations was measured by proficiency scores, patient outcome, and amount of information collected before the first intervention.

Findings.—The nurses' mean proficiency scores were 51% for atrial flutter vs. 35% for ventricular tachycardia. Patient "death" occurred in 13% of atrial flutter and 35% of ventricular tachycardia simulations. Important sources of error included failure to recognize ventricular tachycardia and lack of familiarity with second- and third-line treatments. Of simulations ending in "death," the cause was a medication error in nearly 90% of cases. Treatment was started without obtaining additional data in 48% of ventricular tachycardia and in 28% of the atrial flutter scenarios.

Conclusions.—Critical care nurses must be prepared to make adequate patient assessments and, acting on the relevant cues, accurate decisions. In the present study, nurses had low proficiency scores and poor patient outcomes because of failure to recognize ventricular tachycardia and unfamiliarity with advanced treatments. Clinically, nurses need guidelines for differential diagnosis and treatment until supraventricular tachycardia is definitively diagnosed.

Comments: Say it isn't so. Say that critical care nurses have a better knowledge base than this. This was a sample of critical care nurses with an average of 5 years of experience, 78% of whom held current ACLS certification and medication errors caused 87% of the patient "deaths." What could be the reasons for this? As the authors noted, perhaps results in a simulation are not comparable to those in an actual patient scenario. What was concerning in this study was that nurses did not seek out much information about the patient beyond what was initially provided to them. One hopes that in an actual scenario the nurse would ask for input or verify actions with other colleagues. I think it also is noteworthy that this sample included only 14.8% coronary care unit (CCU) nurses. In most settings, these nurses make the most frequent interpretations of and plan interventions for cardiac dysrhythmias. Perhaps the results would have been different if more CCU nurses had been included in the sample.

Two ongoing clinical problems are highlighted in this study. The first is distinguishing ventricular tachycardia from supraventricular tachycardia. This problem is a major patient care issue. How can we better deal with this and have nurses better prepared to interpret and treat these dysrhythmias correctly? This is a priority for nursing research because it consumes a lot of nursing time and has a dramatic effect on patient outcome. The second problem is how initially to train and then keep nurses current in dysrhythmia recognition and management, especially when they may not deal with it on a frequent basis. Simple didactic content in critical care courses just may not be enough—we need more case studies and mock scenarios to simulate actual conditions more closely.

These data are unacceptable for competent critical care nurses. This article challenges us to rethink our dysrhythmia education and maintenance of ongoing clinical competence in this field. We owe it to our patients.—S. Wingate, RN, DNSc, CCRN, CS

Psychosocial Responses of Patients With Malignant Ventricular Arrhythmias: Assessment and Treatment

Doering L (Cedars Sinai Med Ctr, Los Angeles)

Crit Care Nurse Q 14:72–80, 1991 1–8

Problem.—Progressively more patients are surviving ventricular dysrhythmias and episodes of sudden cardiac death. Psychological distress is increased in patients with cardiac rhythm disorders in general, and in those surviving sudden cardiac death in particular. Anecdotally, many patients are aware of the actual events occurring during resuscitation. The wide range of reactions described in these patients include anxiety with the attendant fear of losing control, depression, denial, and other responses such as dependency conflicts and obsessive-compulsive behavior.

Nursing Interventions.—Most patients require supportive therapy that usually can be initiated by the multidisciplinary health care team (table). The primary goals of treatment are to lessen anxiety and depression and promote effective coping by both the patient and the patient's family. Often the nurse is the first to identify significant symptoms and the one to evaluate supportive measures.

Nursing Implications.—Further study is needed in the following areas: (1) the relationship between neural and psychological mechanisms and the occurrence of ventricular dysrhythmias and sudden cardiac death or malignant dysrhythmias, (3) the effectiveness of various treatment approaches to maladaptive patient responses, and (4) the effect of family interactions on adaptive patient behavior.

Comments: We have witnessed tremendous advances in the pharmacologic and technologic treatment of malignant ventricular dysrhythmias. New antidysrhythmic agents, antitachycardia pacemakers, automatic internal cardioverter-defibrillators, and advanced resuscitation techniques have contributed to enhanced survival in these patients. Less work, however, has been done on the psychosocial aspects of surviving a malignant event and living with

Treatment Approaches for Maladaptive Responses of SCD and HRD Patients

Anxiety
- **Clear information with a hopeful tone**
- **Supportive therapy**
  - **Encourage recollections of events**
  - **Reinforce adaptive denial**
  - **Build coping skills**
  - **Include family members**
- **Pharmacolotherapy**
  - **Benzodiazepams are drugs of choice due to low cardiotoxicity; specific agent should be selected after evaluating symptoms**
  - **ß-Blockers may be used to reduce sympathetic tone**
- **Behavior therapy**
  - **Relaxation response**
  - **Guided imagery and autohypnosis**

Depression
- **Supportive therapy**
  - **Active listening**
  - **Reassurance that the patient has not "failed"**
- **Pharmacotherapy**
  - **Alprazolam has been found to be effective with both adjustment and major depression; has low cardiotoxicity**
  - **Tricyclic antidepressants should be avoided or used with extreme caution**
  - **Second-generation antidepressants (trazodone, maprotiline, amoxapine) may increase ventricular ectopy and should only be used with close monitoring**
  - **If depression is severly disabling or life threatening, carefully controlled ECT may be conisdered when arrhythmia is well controlled**

Abbreviations: SCD, sudden cardiac death; *HRD,* heart rhythm disorders; *ECT,* electroconvulsive therapy.
(Courtesy of Doering L: *Crit Care Nurs* 14:72–80, 1991.)

the treatment(s) for it. Even less has been done on how to intervene to prevent or treat maladaptive coping behaviors in these patients.

Living with the thought of the high risk for a fatal cardiac event truly must be devastating. Indeed, these patients frequently "choose" to invite this very possibility as they undergo repeated electrophysiologic testing. What a dramatic example of the high tech/high touch aspect of critical care nursing—patients are dependent on advanced technology for long-term survival while also requiring supportive interventions to cope with the real possibility of death.

Doering provides an excellent review of the assessment and potential treatment options for patients with malignant ventricular dysrhythmias. She stresses that nurses are the *key* players in the assessment and evaluation of interventions for these patients. But, as Doering noted, most nonpharmacologic interventions for these patients are empiric at this time and have not been validated by scientific inquiry. Wouldn't it be beneficial for critical care nurses to know how to intervene in the early stages to help patients cope with their disease and its treatment? And, one step further, wouldn't it be beneficial for nurses to use proactive, preventive nursing measures to decrease anxiety and depression in this population? This territory is wide open for critical care nurses to investigate.—S. Wingate, RN, DNSc, CCRN, CS

Catheter Ablation of Accessory Atrioventricular Pathways (Wolff-Parkinson-White Syndrome) by Radiofrequency Current

Jackman WM, Wang X, Friday KJ, Roman CA, Moulton KP, Beckman KJ, McClelland JH, Twidale N, Hazlitt HA, Prior MI, Margolis PD, Calame JD, Overholt ED, Lazzara R (Univ of Oklahoma, VA Med Center, Oklahoma City)
N Engl J Med 324:1605–1611, 1991 1–9

Problem.—The definitive treatment for patients with Wolff-Parkinson-White syndrome has been surgical or catheter ablation of accessory pathways using high-energy shocks. An alternative energy source for ablation is radiofrequency current, which produces smaller lesions without adverse effects far from the site where the current is delivered. Catheter techniques for delivering radiofrequency current were explored to reduce the morbidity and mortality associated with accessory-pathway ablation.

Study Methods.—Ablation was tried in 166 patients with 177 accessory pathways. The radiofrequency current was applied through a catheter electrode placed against the mitral or tricuspid annulus or a branch of the coronary sinus. When it was possible, delivery was guided by catheter recordings of accessory-pathway activation.

Findings.—Accessory-pathway conduction was eliminated in 99% of the patients by a median of 3 applications of current. During a mean follow-up of 8 months, 9% of the patients had a return of preexcitation or atrioventricular reentrant tachycardia. All of those patients had a second ablation, which was successful. An electrophysiologic study in 75 patients 3 months after ablation verified that none had accessory-pathway conduction. Three patients had complications from the treatment: atrioventricular block in 1, pericarditis in 1, and cardiac tamponade in 1.

Conclusions.—The results of this study document that catheter delivery of radiofrequency current guided by direct recordings of accessory-pathway activation is very effective for ablating accessory pathways. In this series, there were no deaths, and morbidity was lower than after surgical ablation or catheter ablation with high-energy shocks.

Comments: Patients with Wolff-Parkinson-White syndrome and other problematic paroxysmal supraventricular tachycardias have traditionally undergone open heart surgical procedures and/or long-term antidysrhythmic drug therapy as treatment for their dysrhythmia. Jackman et al. discuss their experiences with a revolutionary treatment technique for these patients—radiofrequency catheter ablation of accessory pathways—and report a very low morbidity, no mortality, and a very high short-term success rate.

Is this procedure part of the new treatment wave for cardiac patients? These patients enter the hospital for an intense few days of high-tech intervention (in this case, catheter ablation and transesophegeal echocardiography [TEE]) and then return home for continued follow-up. The obvious short-term outcomes are a successful procedure with less patient discomfort, shorter hospital stay, a possibly drug-free recovery, and decreased costs. We do not, however, know the long-term effects. Medically, we don't know how patients fare in terms of recurrence of dysrhythmias or symptoms. Psychosocially, we don't know how patients fare in terms of anxiety levels and quality of life.

This procedure has considerable implications for critical care nursing practice. First, in a limited period of time, these patients must be prepared for the electrophysiologic study as well as the very lengthy ablation procedure. Second, they then require very close observation as they recover from this procedure and also undergo other diagnostic tests such as TEE. Third, patients need critical assessments of their cardiac rhythm. The potential need for a temporary (and then perhaps permanent) pacemaker is high because of damage to the AV node. Fourth, these patients require strong psychosocial support because they may have very high anxiety levels resulting from a prolonged disease course and/or prior unsuccessful therapeutic procedures.

As critical care nurses, we welcome a procedure with the potential benefits that this one has for the patient. But we also must develop nursing plans of care for short-stay, high-risk patients needing concentrated assessment, educational, and psychosocial interventions.—S. Wingate, RN, DNSc, CCRN, CS

Acute Myocardial Ischemia

Outcome of Patients Who Were Admitted to a New Short-Stay Unit to "Rule-Out" Myocardial Infarction

Gaspoz J-M, Lee TH, Cook EF, Weisberg MC, Goldman L (Brigham and Women's Hosp; Harvard School of Public Health, Boston)
Am J Cardiol 68:145–149, 1991 1–10

Problem.—As many as 70% of patients in the coronary care unit are admitted to rule out myocardial infarction. One approach to correcting this problem would be to have a cost-effective alternative to the coronary unit for those whose likelihood of having an infarct is low to moderate.

Methods.—A 2-bed nonintensive, short-stay coronary observation unit was established within a 10-bed holding unit adjacent to the emergency room. The unit, with telemetric monitoring equipment, admitted patients whose probability of acute infarction was no greater than 10% and who were expected to stay no longer than 48 hours. Those admitted did not require more than the available degree of nursing care. The nurse/patient ratio was 1:5, with at least 1 nurse experienced in interpreting cardiac monitoring tracings always physically present in the holding ar-

Clinical Characteristics of the 512 Admissions to the Coronary Observation Unit

		No. (%)
Male gender		247 (48%)
Age (yr) (mean ± SD)		59 ± 15
Chief complaint:		
Chest pain		488 (95%)
Arm, neck, epigastric pain		24 (5%)
Among those with chest pain	(n = 488)	
Chest pain of substernal location	354 (73%)	
Quality of chest pain		
Pressure	312 (64%)	
Sharp	51(10%)	
Other	125 (26%)	
Chest pain reproduced by		
Deep breathing	28 (6%)	
Palpation	40 (8%)	
Position	20 (4%)	
Time since onset of suspected cardiac ischemic pain		
≤4 hours		223 (45%)
4–12 hours		115 (23%)
>12 hours		162 (32%)
Duration of longest episode of pain		
≤60 minutes		231 (51%)
>60 minutes		223 (49%)
History of angina or myocardial infarction		224 (44%)
Associated symptoms		
Diaphoresis		137 (27%)
Dyspnea		210 (41%)
Dizziness		58 (11%)
Physical examination: > bibasilar rales		71 (14%)
Emergency room electrocardiogram		
Changes consistent with ischemia or infarction not known to be old		84 (16%)
Changes consistent with ischemia or infarction known to be old		73 (14%)
Other old or new abnormalities		97 (19%)
Nonspecific ST-T-wave changes		161 (32%)
Normal		97 (19%)

Note: Missing data: time since onset of pain, 12 observations; duration of longest episode of pain, 58 observations.

(Courtesy of Gaspoz J-M, Lee TH, Cook EF, et al: *Am J Cardiol* 68:145–149, 1991.)

eas. The ECGs were recorded every 12 hours, and the serum creatine kinase and its MB isoenzyme were estimated at admission and then every 8 hours for the first 24 hours. All patients discharged from the coronary observation unit were evaluated for the ability to ambulate, but only 19% underwent formal stress testing.

Findings.—Of 512 patients admitted to the new unit, all but 5% had a chief complaint of chest pain (table). Acute myocardial infarction was diagnosed in 15 instances (3%), most often from the ECG and enzymatic findings in the first 24 hours. Eighty-three percent of the patients were discharged home directly from the coronary observation unit, and only 1 of them—after leaving against medical advice—had an acute myocardial infarction. One fourth of these patients had acute ischemic heart disease without infarction.

Conclusions.—The idea of a precoronary care area was suggested by Lown et al. in 1969 but was not developed until now. It usually takes less than 24 hours to rule out myocardial infarction, and most complications occur during this period. Short-stay coronary observation units are safe and adequate for ruling out acute myocardial infarction in a select group of cardiac patients who have a low probability of myocardial infarction.

Comments: Patients with acute myocardial infarction (AMI) who are improperly sent home from the emergency department (ED) have a significantly higher mortality than do those admitted to the coronary care unit (CCU) (1). Patients with a low probability of AMI (< 5% to 10%) represent a select subgroup in which the probability is too low to warrant a CCU admission to be cost-effective. Yet, the probability of AMI in such patients is significant enough to make discharge from the ED dangerous. Thus, such patients may benefit from admission to a short-stay coronary observation unit with monitoring and resuscitation equipment but without the other expensive services provided by a CCU or telemetry unit. It is essential, however, that such units be adequately staffed with nursing personnel who are certified in both basic and advanced cardiac life support and who have expertise in interpreting cardiac dysrhythmias. Strict criteria must be developed for transfer to the CCU should patients develop complications and require more intensive therapy and surveillance.

It is important to note, however, that the 6- to 24-month prognosis of patients hospitalized with acute ischemic pain but no AMI is similar to that of patients with AMI (2). Almost a quarter of the patients in this study were discharged home from the coronary observation unit with the diagnosis of acute ischemic heart disease. Moreover, 5 of these patients developed AMI within 3 days of their discharge. Thus, early discharge from short-stay units may be premature in some patients who are at high risk for developing complications shortly thereafter.

The nursing implications are clear. Patients must be made aware of the necessity for immediate cardiology follow-up with expedient exercise stress testing. Although stress testing is not flawless in diagnosing coronary artery disease, it is valuable in estimating prognosis. In addition, patients must understand that continued or recurring symptoms must be evaluated immediately. Patients and families must receive adequate information regarding signs and symptoms of AMI, what to do, and how to seek medical attention without delay. They must be taught to take their new medications, including nitroglycerin, properly, and they need to know exactly what to do if the nitroglycerin does not provide relief from pain. Any guilt or hesitancy about returning to the ED must be discussed. Short-stay coronary observation units provide exciting possibilities in reducing health care costs, but they also present nurses with many patient teaching challenges.—C.E. Guzzetta, RN, PhD, FAAN

References

1. Lee TH, Juarez G, Cook EF, et al: Ruling out acute myocardial infarction. A prospective multicenter validation of a 12-hour strategy for patients at low risk. *N Engl J Med* 324:1239–1246, 1991.
2. Schroeder JS, Lamb IH, Hu M: Do patients in whom myocardial infarction has been ruled out have a better prognosis after hospitalization than those surviving infarction? *N Engl J Med* 303:1–5, 1980.

Is Coronary-Care-Unit Admission Restricted for Elderly Patients? A Multicenter Study

Fleming C, D'Agostino RB, Selker HP (New England Med Ctr Hosps, Boston)
Am J Public Health 81:1121–1126, 1991 1–11

Problem.—In an environment of increasing health care costs, the appropriateness of unrestricted high technology care for elderly patients has been questioned. One report suggested that the threshold for critical care unit admission is already age-related, with fewer elderly patients admitted despite their more severe disease. To test this assertion, the effect of age on likelihood of coronary care unit (CCU) admission for patients with acute myocardial infarction was investigated.

Study Methods.—The study sample was comprised of 3,225 patients at 6 hospitals; data were collected as part of a prospective study of CCU admitting practices. For analysis, patients were stratified by age, with pa-

Physicians' Triage Disposition for Patients With Acute Myocardial Infarction by Age Groups

Age (years)	Patients Admitted to CCU n (%)	Patients Not Admitted to CCU n (%)	Relative Risk CCU Nonadmission (95% CI)
40-74	557 (90)	63 (10)	1.0
75-79	69 (79)	18 (21)	2.09 (1.16,3.37)
80-84	50 (81)	12 (19)	2.18 (1.09,4.36)
85+	27 (66)	14 (34)	4.25 (2.10,8.59)

Note: Relative risks are adjusted for admitting hospital and compare rates of CCU nonadmission for older age groups to those of patients in the 40–74 year age group.

(Courtesy of Fleming C, D'Agostino RB, Selker HP: *Am J Public Health* 81:1121–1126, 1991.)

tients 75 years of age or older considered elderly. The main outcome measure was the patients' probability of not being admitted to the CCU. Twenty-four percent of the study sample was considered elderly.

Findings.—The likelihood of CCU nonadmission increased with advancing age (table). Elderly patients were 2.5 times less likely to be admitted to the CCU than were younger patients. This was the case even in patients whose admission diagnosis was myocardial infarction or "rule-out myocardial infarction." These differences in CCU admission were not explained by any apparent differences in the patients' clinical presentations. Mortality was lower in younger than in elderly patients, but was similar for elderly patients admitted to the CCU vs. those admitted to the wards or sent home.

Conclusions.—Emergency room physicians appear to restrict CCU admission for elderly patients with acute myocardial infarction. These differences do not result from misdiagnosis in the emergency department. More studies are needed of elderly patients in other critical care settings and with other conditions.

Comments: Another chapter on the issue of access to health care. However, this unequal access to health care appears to be the result of age and not of money or insurance. Unfortunately, this is not an isolated study. Montague et al. (1), in a study of practice patterns in acute myocardial infarction, found that patients older than 70 years had markedly higher mortality and less aggressive medical management than did younger patients. Are older patients at higher risk for increased mortality because they haven't been given equal access to therapies or because their age or disease simply puts them at higher risk? We don't know, but as Fleming et al. noted, aren't these higher risk older patients *precisely the ones* who need access to the CCU and to aggressive medical management? In fact, might they need it even more than the lower risk patient?

It is recognized that several important areas were not evaluated in this study; that is, *why* were these triage decisions made, and what was the effect on the quality of patients' lives? Despite these unknowns, the nursing implications of this study are significant. Do we advocate equal care for patients regardless of age? Do we question seemingly unusual triage decisions? More importantly, do we have our own biases about care for the elderly? If the trend continues for increased numbers of elderly patients with chronic diseases, how will we balance the quality issues with the access and treatment issues? Is care for the elderly in CCU cost-effective? How do we *know* that the high tech, high-cost care in a CCU pays off in improved patient outcomes for elderly myocardial infarction patients? How do we know it *doesn't?*—S. Wingate, RN, DNSc, CCRN, CS

Reference

1. Montague TJ, Ikuta RM, Wong RY, et al: Comparison of risk and patterns of practice in patients older and younger than 70 years with acute myocardial infarction in a two-year period (1987-1989). *Am J Cardiol* 68:843–847, 1991.

Treatment-Seeking Behavior Among Those With Signs and Symptoms of Acute Myocardial Infarction

Dracup K, Moser DK (Univ of California, Los Angeles)

Heart Lung 20:570–575, 1991 1–12

Problem.—Significant delays in seeking medical care for the symptoms of acute myocardial infarction may hinder the physician's ability to limit infarct size or may result in mortality. Thrombolysis has a 4-hour "window of opportunity," but 26% to 44% of patients delay longer than 4 hours in seeking medical attention. Delay in treatment-seeking behavior of patients with symptoms of AMI was examined to identify characteristics associated with prolonged response time.

Study Methods.—More than 12 published research studies spanning 20 years were analyzed and variables associated with increased or reduced delay were enumerated.

Findings.—The 6 commonly recognized phases of delay are outlined in Table 1. Comparison of variables contributing to prehospital delay time across studies is difficult because of methodologic differences and study limitations, but some conclusions are possible. Variables associated with decreased delay times are pain recognized as cardiac in origin, hemodynamic instability, severe chest pain, younger age, and consultation

TABLE 1.—Categorization of Delay Time in the Treatment of Acute Myocardial Infarction

Prodromal Period: period between the initial awareness of a health deviation and the onset of acute symptoms.

Definition Period: period of self-evaluation that occurs between the onset of acute symptoms and the seeking of lay advice.

Lay Consultation Period: period between seeking lay advice and medical consultation. In one study of more than 1,100 patients, 93% sought lay advice.

Medical Consultation Period: interval between calling a physician or other source of medical care and traveling to the hospital.

Travel Period: time spent traveling to the hospital. This time period is insignificant with respect to total delay time.

Hospital Procedural Period: time spent in the hospital emergency room or in the admission office before treatment begins.

(Adapted from Dracup K, Moser DK: *Heart Lung* 20:570–575, 1991.)

TABLE 2.—Extent of Delay From AMI Symptom Onset to Thrombolytic Therapy

Patient delay	• Median delay of 2-4 hr • Longest component of treatment delay • Difficult to decrease
EMS delay	• <50% use by patients with suspected AMI • EMS identification of patients with AMI decreases time to treatment • Prehospital thrombolytic therapy is feasible
Hospital delay	• Average delay of 84 min from hospital arrival to thrombolytic treatment

(Courtesy of Ho MT: *Heart Lung* 20:566–9, 1991.)

with a co-worker. Variables associated with increased delay times are a medical history of chronic disease, older age, black race, seeking advice from a physician or family member, symptom onset on a weekday, or attempts at self-treatment. Socioeconomic status and educational level do not affect delay time.

Recommendations.—Individuals who are older than age 65 years; are black; or have a history of angina, diabetes, or hypertension should receive particular education in differentiating cardiac symptoms from their symptoms of chronic disease and accessing the emergency medical system. Public educational campaigns should emphasize the importance of a quick decision to seek medical care. Unfortunately, experience with

TABLE 3.—Components of Delay From AMI Symptom Onset to Thrombolytic Therapy

Patient delay	• Total delay = Appraisal delay + Illness delay + utilization delay
EMS delay	• Nonuse • Delay from EMS call to paramedic arrival • On-scene time • Transport time
Hospital delay	• Identification of patients with suspected AMI • Awaiting laboratory tests results and electrocardiogram • Obtaining cardiologic consultation • Obtaining thrombolytic agent from pharmacy • Transfer to coronary care unit

(Courtesy of Ho MT: *Heart Lung* 20:566–9, 1991.)

some public educational campaigns has shown that increased awareness does not change behavior. Consultation with a private physician increased delay; the public must be informed that the best course of action in the case of cardiac symptoms is seeking emergency medical care immediately. Physicians can hold in-service classes for cardiac patients and instruct their staff to tell patients with cardiac symptoms to go to the hospital immediately. Family members and other potential witnesses must be educated to "take charge" when an individual experiences cardiac symptoms. The nurses' contribution includes special education and reinforcement for spouses or family members in differentiating symptoms and seeking treatment and in preparing for a cardiac emergency by learning cardiopulmonary resuscitation skills.

Comments: Although delay in seeking treatment for acute myocardial infarction (AMI) is not a new problem, the current era of reperfusion therapy has heightened the perilous nature of this problem. In this comprehensive article, Dracup and Moser synthesize the results of studies on delay time conducted over the past 20 years. The purpose of this review was to identify factors that contribute to patient indecision so that intervention might be developed and tested to reduce delay time. This review solidly isolates one startling trend—that there has been little improvement in reducing prehospital delay time over the past 3 decades.

Delay time involves the amount of time that elapses between onset of AMI symptoms and the initiation of definitive therapy in the hospital. Dracup and Moser have conceptualized this delay time into 6 phases (Table 1). In contrast, Ho has conceptualized 3 phases of delay time (Table 2 and Table 3) (1). What is clear from these tables is that the most significant chunk of the total delay time is attributed to the time it takes patients to decide that they are ill enough to seek medical attention.

In the past, the delay problem has been studied using the medical model that focuses on the patient's demographic and clinical characteristics as predictors of delay. Patients then were categorized as high or low risk for delay. Dracup and Moser argue that this model is flawed because it places the blame for delay solely on the patient and it does not provide direction for developing comprehensive intervention programs. Thus they suggest that this old problem be attacked from a new prospective. They recommend the use of an interaction model to study delay problems. This includes the critical role that other people play in the patient's decision-making process.

As I read the article, I had a sudden intuitive feeling that maybe Dracup and Moser were right. Maybe we haven't been effective in reducing delay times over the past 30 years because we have been concentrating on the wrong variables. For example, if we educate patients about the signs and symptoms of AMI and the need to seek prompt medical treatment, we have increased their knowledge, but we have not changed their behavior in terms of using the emergency medical system (EMS) and in reducing delay times. Thus, maybe we need to bridge this knowledge-behavior gap and focus on the interactional roles of others and the emotional as well as cognitive implications for delay for all those involved. This interactional framework then could provide the direction for future interventions that focus specifically on the following:

- teaching that focuses on individuals at high risk for delays
- educational campaigns that focus on the importance of seeking immediate medical care and emphasize problem-solving techniques and fundamental steps that need to be taken when symptoms occur. The use of denial as a contributing factor in delay time needs additional study.
- teaching that emphasizes the use of the EMS. Because only half of the patients suspected of AMI use the EMS, the public needs to understand and be reassured that a heart attack is an emergency that justifies the use of the EMS. Teaching should address the emotional and cognitive reasons that persons refrain from calling the EMS, such as fear or embarrassment, concerns for inappropriately using the EMS when patients judge that their symptoms do not warrant its use, and rationalization that self-transport seems faster or is more appropriate.
- teaching that focuses on family members and emphasizes their need to assume responsibility for the decision-making process. Most persons experience symptoms of AMI in the presence of family members. Family members may be motivated to share the patient's denial or may be less willing to confront the patient's delay than a co-worker or stranger. Thus, teaching must target family members and must stress the critical nature of their role and the need to act independently and quickly.

If we haven't made any progress in changing delay time in the past 30 years, then perhaps we have been asking the wrong questions. The time has come to confront this problem from a new perspective.—C.E. Guzzetta, RN, PhD, FAAN

References

1. Ho, MT: Delays in the treatment of acute myocardial infarction: An overview. *Heart Lung* 20:566–569, 1991.
2. Alonzo, AA: Acute illness behavior: A conceptual exploration and specification. *Soc Sci Med* 14:515–526, 1980.

Depression and Type A Behavior Pattern in Patients With Coronary Artery Disease: Relationships to Painful Versus Silent Myocardial Ischemia and β-Endorphin Responses During Exercise

Light KC, Herbst MC, Bragdon EE, Hinderliter AL, Koch GG, Davis MR, Sheps DS (Univ of North Carolina at Chapel Hill)
Psychosom Med 53:669–683, 1991 1–13

Problem.—Myocardial ischemia does not always produce pain. Even in patients who have had recurrent angina, silent ischemic episodes may be much more frequent than painful episodes. Depressed mood correlates with chronic pain, and patients with coronary artery disease who have high depression scores may report more anginal pain during exercise-induced myocardial ischemia. In at least some patients, exercise-induced pain may be suppressed by increased release of β-endorphin. In this study, the relationship between depression and the reporting of anginal pain and β-endorphin levels during exercise-induced myocardial ischemia was determined. The relationship between type A vs. type B behavior patterns and the reporting of pain and β-endorphin levels was also evaluated.

Study Methods.—Forty-five patients with coronary artery disease underwent exercise testing to evoke myocardial ischemia. The Minnesota Multiphasic Personality Inventory depression scale was used to assess depressed mood, and type A and type B behavior were evaluated by the structured interview. Pain measures included the time of onset of pain and the severity of pain measured on a visual analogue scale. Plasma β-endorphins were measured at baseline and at the end of exercise.

Findings.—All patients had ST-segment depression during exercise, but only 18 (40%) reported anginal pain. Patients with higher depression scores were more likely to experience angina and rated their pain as more severe than those who had lower depression scores. In addition, patients with higher depression scores had less marked rises in plasma β-endorphin levels. Hemodynamic responses to exercise were similar in the 2 groups. Type A vs. type B behavior did not correlate with greater anginal pain or changes in β-endorphin levels.

Implications.—Patients who have ischemic heart disease who are also depressed tend to have blunted β-endorphin responses to exercise as well as more marked pain. It is not clear whether more intense pain enhances depressive mood in these patients or whether preexisting depression alters endocrine and β-endorphin responses to enhance anginal pain. In any case, depressive symptoms in patients with coronary artery disease deserve close attention.

Comments: The quest has only begun to determine the precise mechanism responsible for why some patients with myocardial ischemia do not develop chest pain. Silent myocardial ischemia is present when there is objective evidence of myocardial ischemia (e.g., transient ST-segment changes, myocardial perfusion defects, or reversible regional wall motions abnormalities [1]), but without the presence of chest pain or other anginal equivalents (2). Silent myocardial ischemia occurs much more frequently than painful myocardial ischemia in patients with coronary artery disease.

Many theories have been offered about why some ischemic episodes are painless. It has been proposed that myocardial ischemia involves a series of steps, with chest pain being the last step in the ischemic sequence (1). Thus, silent ischemic episodes may progress to objective phases (e.g., electrocardiographic changes) but fail to reach the pain threshold. Likewise, it has been suggested that silent episodes may be less severe and may not last as long as symptomatic episodes in the same patient (3). Some researchers have proposed that psychological and cultural factors are responsible for changing pain perception (1). Still others have suggested that patients may have a defective perception of painful stimuli or may have a higher threshold for pain (1,3).

In this study, Light and colleagues have done an excellent job of building on the positive results of previous studies. The role of psychological and behavioral factors (i.e., depression and type A vs. type B behavior patterns) and the role of altered pain transmission (i.e., by β-endorphin levels) have been investigated. The central findings demonstrate that depressed patients respond to exercise with lowered β-endorphin levels and enhanced reporting of anginal pain. In my mind, this study does more to establish the role of why people *do* develop chest pain with myocardial ischemia than it does to explain why they *do not.* Nevertheless, it points out some important nursing implications: patients who are clinically depressed must be carefully assessed and referred to the appropriate resources for psychological, behavioral, and pharmacologic therapy aimed at relieving depression and enhancing coping skills.

Although the findings from this study are sound, they cannot be generalized to all patients who experience painless episodes of myocardial ischemia. They do not explain, for example, the coexistence of symptomatic and silent episodes of myocardial ischemia in the same individual. It is likely that different psychophysiologic mechanisms for silent myocardial ischemia exist in different individuals. Clearly the answers are not all in. The quest continues. Keep an eye out for the answers in the future.—C.E. Guzzetta, RN, PhD, FAAN

References

1. Deedwania PC, Carbajal EV: Silent myocardial ischemia: A clinical perspective. *Arch Intern Med* 151: 2373–2382, 1991.
2. Parnley W: Prevalence and clinical significance of myocardial ischemia. *Circulation* 80(suppl 4): 68–73, 1989.
3. Valle GA, Lemberg L: Silent ischemia: A clinical update. *Chest* 97:186–191, 1990.

Circadian Variations in Myocardial Ischemia: Implications for Management

Pepine CJ (VA Med Ctr, Gainesville, Fla)

JAMA 265:386–390, 1991 — 1–14

Problem.—Although myocardial ischemic activity can occur at any time, between 6 AM and noon circadian peaks as high as twofold and threefold above baseline activity occur in myocardial ischemia (Fig 1–4), acute myocardial infarction, stroke, and sudden death. In the 2% to 4% of patients with variant angina, this peak is shifted to the very early morning hours. Circadian variations in myocardial ischemia and their implications for management were discussed.

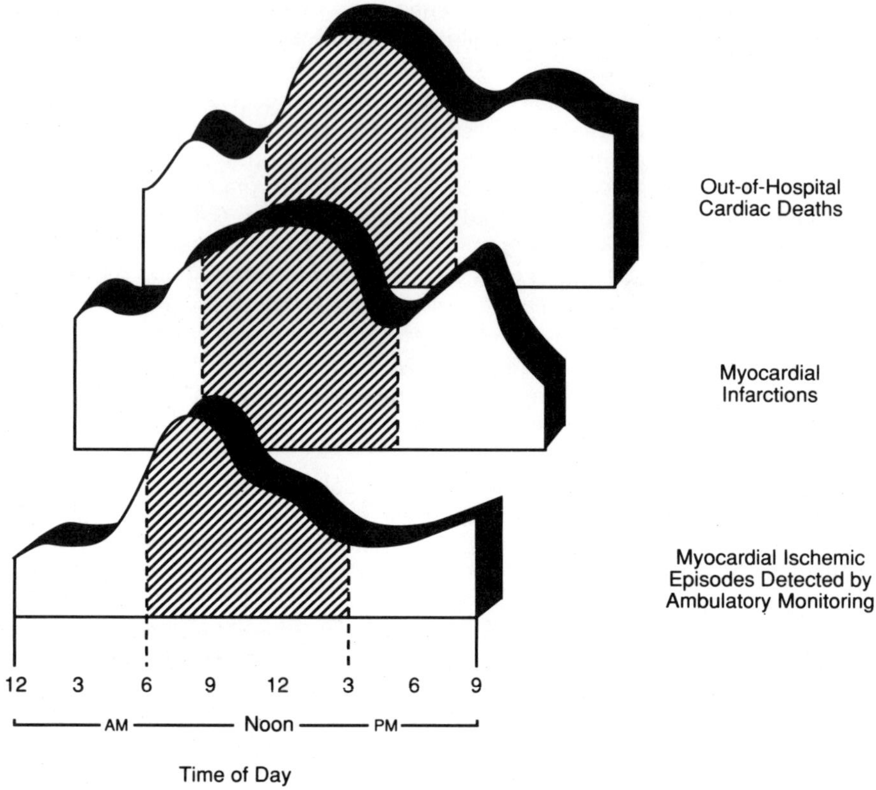

Fig 1–4.—The relative distribution of myocardial ischemic episodes detected by ambulatory monitoring (*bottom*), myocardial infarctions (*center*), and out-of-hospital cardiac deaths (*top*). The peak frequencies in all 3 conditions occur after the patient awakens in the morning and remain elevated until midafternoon. (Modified from Rocco et al) (Courtesy of Pepine CJ: *JAMA* 265:386–390, 1991.)

Treatment Implications.—Because of the circadian peak in ischemic episodes, a long-acting nitrate preparation should be taken on awakening. Its rapid onset of action will provide protection within minutes against the surge in ischemic activity that begins after awakening. A nitrate-free period to reduce the likelihood of tolerance development would be best from about 10 PM to 8 AM, while the patient is asleep. The increase in ischemic activity that occurs just after waking is eliminated by β-blockers. The dosing schedule should be designed so that adequate tissue levels of the receptor blocker are present when the patient awakens. Dosing at night with a long-acting β-blocker should provide optimal antiischemic protection between awakening and noon. Calcium antagonists effectively reduce ischemia but not heart rate and do not seem to change the circadian distribution of ischemia. Heart-rate–active calcium antagonists may slightly modify the circadian distribution of ischemia, however.

Nursing Implications.—Health care professionals must give attention to the vulnerable morning period when choosing and timing medications. Consideration of circadian variations in myocardial ischemia may prevent or reduce ischemia and modify potential disease-triggering maechanisms.

Comments: You may be a klutz on the dance floor, but you have rhythm. Indeed, you have numerous biological rhythms that dance in synchronous harmony with the rhythm of nature. Should you get "out of step," dysynchrony and illness will ensue. Knowledge of circadian rhythms has been accumulating for more than 2,000 years, when Hippocrates first suggested that regularity of body functions was a sign of health. Research in the field of chronobiology has yielded surprising data. Circadian variations have been discovered for many bodily functions, such as cognitive performance, sensory ability, pain perception, allergic responses, drug elimination, response to toxins, mood, sleep-wake cycles, thermoregulation, fluid and electrolyte balance, and cardiovascular performance. Despite these findings, medical researchers have given little heed to chronobiological influences. Recently studies of circadian variations in cardiovascular function, published in "mainstream" medical journals, are finally arousing interest in this important issue.

Pepine's review article nicely illustrates the circadian pattern of myocardial ischemic episodes. These episodes are apparently related to lower blood fibrinolytic activity, higher platelet aggregability, and increased plasma catecholamine levels found in the morning (1). Knowledge of this pathologic rhythmicity enables the clinician to anticipate myocardial and cerebral ischemic events and possibly prevent their occurrences (i.e., appropriately timed administration of nitrates or β-blockers in myocardial ischemia).

Nurses have not kept pace with the field of chronobiology, despite the profound influence of circadian rhythms on their performance and their patients' response to therapy. We need more research related to circadian rhythms and the critically ill patient: an investigation of optimal times for medication administration and for collection of laboratory specimens; a comparison of fluctuations in physiologic functions (temperature, blood pressure, pulse, and urine output) in the elderly patient with that of the younger patient; and determination of optimal scheduling of nurses' shift work to maintain maximum chronobiological synchrony. We also must reexamine the critical care environment. It is known that our circadian rhythms are synchronized by outside triggers such as light-dark and sleep-wake cycles. How do we ensure an environment that maintains the patient's chronobiologic integrity? We must first be attuned to our patient's inner rhythm and stay in step with it by appropriately darkening the room and allowing clear rest-sleep cycles whenever possible. It is time we stop "dancing to a different drummer."—C. Kessler, RN, MN, CCRN, CS

Reference

1. Panza JA, Epstein SE, Quyyumi AA: Circadian variation in vascular tone and its relation to alpha-sympathetic vasoconstrictor activity. *N Engl J Med* 325:986–990, 1991.

Prognostic Importance of Delayed Q-Wave Evolution 3 to 24 Hours After Initiation of Thrombolytic Therapy for Acute Myocardial Infarction

Eisenberg MJ, Barbash GI, Hod H, Roth A, Shachar A, Zolti L, Rabinowitz B, Kaplinsky E, Laniado S, Modan M (Univ of California at San Francisco; Sheba Med Ctr, Tel Hashomer, Israel; Tel Aviv Med Ctr)

Am J Cardiol 67:231–235, 1991 1–15

Problem.—Although many studies have shown the prognostic value of Q waves after acute myocardial infarction, most studies were done before thrombolytic therapy became widespread.

Study Methods.—The timing of Q-wave development and its prognostic importance were examined in 201 patients given thrombolytic treatment for a first acute myocardial infarction. Seventy percent of the patients had evidence of Q-wave infarction within 3 hours of the start of thrombolytic treatment, and another 16% had Q waves after 3 hours but before discharge. No Q waves developed in 14% of patients before discharge.

Findings.—When Q waves were delayed (after 3 hours), patients had lower peak creatine kinase levels and better left ventricular function than did those with early Q-wave infarction. In addition, patients with delayed or no Q waves had better ejection fractions and less evidence of heart failure at the time of discharge than did those with early Q waves. There were no significant differences between the early and delayed groups with regard to age, gender, or infarct site. The early appearance of Q waves correlated with higher hospital mortality, although this was not statistically significant. The 1-year mortality was similar in both groups.

Conclusions.—Patients with acute myocardial infarction in whom Q waves appear more than 3 hours after the onset are clinically and prognostically similar to those having non–Q-wave infarction. In addition to stratifying patients according to the presence or absence of Q waves, it appears helpful to specify when Q waves develop.

Comments: To the West Coast surfer, Q waves might signify an "awesome" new form of oceanic rollercoaster to challenge with a surfboard and skill. To cardiac nurses, Q waves are myocardial tombstones, signifying cellular necrosis. Their appearance is worrisome. Past studies suggest that the exact timing of their appearance is also significant, at least in terms of in-hospital morbidity and mortality (1). Yet in this era of thrombolysis, is the timing of Q-wave development as significant?

In their study, Eisenberg et al. have demonstrated that early Q-wave development (from the onset of myocardial infarction to 3 hours postinfusion of thrombolytic agents) is associated with increased in-hospital mortality and ventricular dysfunction. This is a reasonable finding because the appearance of Q waves depends on the amount and site of myocardial necrosis. A more intriguing finding is that patients with delayed Q-wave development (> 3 hours postinfusion of thrombolytics) have outcomes similar to those with non–Q-wave infarctions. The reason for this is not quite clear. Delayed Q-wave development could signify an incomplete infarction or a lower grade coronary occlusion and increased collateralization. Perhaps thrombolytic intervention curtails the process of myocardial necrosis, resulting in slower Q-wave evolution. It would be interesting to know whether the phenomenon of delayed Q-wave development occurs more often in patients receiving thrombolytic therapy. For this reason, more study in this area is required.

Why should nurses care about the timing of Q-wave evolution? For the same reason that differentiating between inferior and anterior myocardial infarctions is important: to be more prepared for specific, potential complications. So, if your patient develops an early Q wave, be prepared for a rough ride. If the Q wave is late in developing, just "hang 10" and let your patient ride "the wave."—C. Kessler, RN, MN, CCRN, CS

Reference

1. Maisel AS, Ahnave S, Gilpin E, et al: Prognosis after extension of myocardial infarct: The role of Q-wave and non-Q-wave infarction. *Circulation* 71:211–217, 1985.

Effect of Age on Use of Thrombolytic Therapy and Mortality in Acute Myocardial Infarction

Weaver WD, Litwin PE, Martin JS, Kudenchuk PJ, Maynard C, Eisenberg MS, Ho MT, Cobb LA, Kennedy JW, Wirkus MS (MITI Project Group, Seattle, Wash)

J Am Coll Cardiol 18:657–662, 1991 1–16

Problem.—Several studies suggest that thrombolytic treatment lowers mortality in selected patients suspected of having acute myocardial infarction, and that it may be most effective in the elderly. However, only a small proportion of patients studied have been elderly.

Study Methods.—Age-related outcomes were reviewed in a series of 3,256 consecutive patients hospitalized for acute myocardial infarction as part of the Myocardial Infarction Triage and Intervention (MITI) Project. Fifty-six percent of the group were over age 65 years and 28% were age 75 and older.

Age-Related Findings.—Prior angina, hypertension, and heart failure were all more prevalent in older patients. Systemic thrombolysis was attempted in 29% of patients less than 75 years old and in 5% of older patients. It was estimated that no more than 15% of patients age 75 or older were suitable candidates for thrombolytic treatment. Unexpected

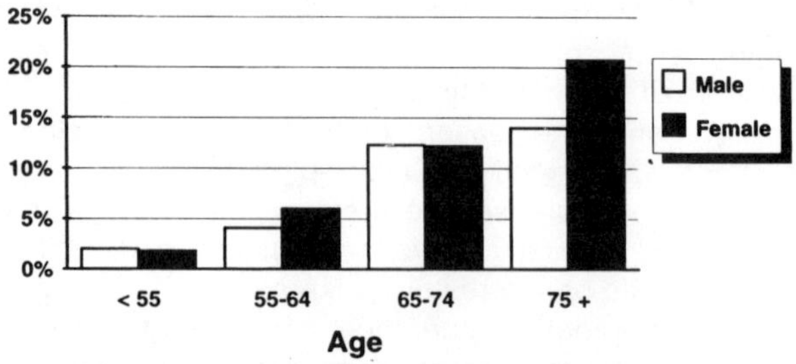

Fig 1–5.—Mortality rates by age for the 3,256 patients with acute myocardial infarction. No patient <47 years of age died during hospitalization, whereas the overall mortality rate in patients ≥75 years was 18%. Gender-specific mortality rates were similar in all but the last stratum. The median age of men and women in the group ≥75 years of age was 80 and 82 years, respectively. Age adjusted mortality rates for men and women were not significantly different (9.1% and 11.3%, respectively). (Courtesy of Weaver WD, Litwin PE, Martin JS, et al: *J Am Coll Cardiol* 18:657–662, 1991.)

cardiac arrest occurred less frequently in older patients, but stroke occurred substantially more often with advancing age (3.9% of elderly patients compared with 1.2% of those 65 years of age or less). Hospital mortality rose with advancing age (Fig 1–5). The 2 factors statistically associated with the risk of death, heart failure, or reinfarction were past heart failure and increasing age (table).

Implications.—Elderly patients often have acute infarction in a setting of past complications from ischemic heart disease, and they have a very high hospital mortality rate. More needs to be learned about the efficacy of both pharmacologic and mechanical means of reperfusion in the elderly.

Comment: *See comment after Abstract 1–17.*

Clinical Event Rates (%) During Hospitalization by Age Strata

	Age (years)					
	<55	55–64	65–74	≥75	All	p Value*
Cardiac arrest	4.1	2.9	1.8	1.2	2.4	0.001
Heart failure	15	24	31	31	26	<0.0001
Stroke	1.4	1.2	2	3.9	2.2	0.0004
Transfusion	8	12	18	12	13	<0.0001
Reinfarction	2.6	2.5	6.2	5.5	4.4	0.0001
Death	2	4.6	12.3	17.8	10	<0.0001

*p values are for chi-square tests with 3 degrees of freedom.
(Courtesy of Weaver WD, Litwin PE, Martin JS, et al: *J Am Coll Cardiol* 18:657–662, 1991.)

Thrombolytic Therapy in Patients Requiring Cardiopulmonary Resuscitation

Tenaglia AN, Califf RM, Candela RJ, Kereiakes DJ, Berrios E, Young SY, Stack RS, Topol EJ (Duke Univ, Durham, NC; Riverside Methodist Hosp, Columbus, Ohio; Christ Hosp, Cincinnati; Univ of Michigan, Ann Arbor)

Am J Cardiol 68:1015–1019, 1991 1–17

Problem.—It has been suggested that cardiopulmonary resuscitation (CPR) is a contraindication to thrombolytic therapy. However, there have been no studies specifically addressing this question, and patients requiring CPR might benefit most from thrombolysis. Patients from the Thrombolysis and Angioplasty in Myocardial Infarction trials who did receive CPR were compared with those who did not.

Study Methods.—The trials included 708 consecutive patients with signs of myocardial infarction, 59 of whom required less than 10 minutes of CPR before, or had CPR within, 6 hours of receiving lytic therapy. Patients who needed more than 10 minutes of CPR were excluded from the trial. Baseline characteristics, including sex, coronary artery disease risk factors, and time until treatment, were similar between the 2 groups.

Findings.—Seventy-three percent of patients required CPR for ventricular fibrillation and 24% for ventricular tachycardia. Resuscitation lasted a median of only 1 minute; the 25th percentile of duration was also 1 minute, and the 75th percentile was 5 minutes. A median of 2 cardioversions/defibrillations were required. The CPR group were significantly more likely to have anterior infarctions, to have an infarct related to the left anterior descending artery, and to have lower ejection fractions on their initial ventriculograms. In-hospital mortalities were 12% for the CPR group vs. 6% for the non-CPR group; most common causes of death were pump failure and dysrhythmias in the former group and pump failure and reinfarction in the latter. No bleeding complications were directly attributable to CPR; the 2 groups had similar decreases in hematocrit and need for transfusion.

Conclusions.—Thrombolytic therapy appears to cause no additional complications in myocardial infarction patients who have received less than 10 minutes of CPR. Thus such therapy should not be contraindicated by CPR, particularly of short duration. In fact, these patients appear to represent a high-risk group who can benefit greatly from lytic therapy.

Comments: In this era of thrombolytic therapy for coronary artery occlusion, many of us have developed a rather smug attitude with regard to early treatment of acute myocardial infarction. Gone are the days when a little morphine, oxygen, and lidocaine were all that pharmacologically could be offered to the patient while we simply watched and waited for the myocardial infarction to go through its evolutionary stages. Now we have a cadre of thrombolytic agents—"silver bullets"—to shoot at deadly clots with remarkable accuracy. Unfortunately, this heart-saving therapy is prohibited for some patients who need it most.

Weaver et al. (Abstract 1–16) examined the use of thrombolytic therapy in the elderly population as part of an ambitious registry of patients with myocardial infarction. While it has been acknowledged that thrombolytic therapy reduces the mortality rate in the elderly, only 5% of patients over 75 years of age received thrombolytic treatment. It is interesting to note that 15% of these patients were actually suitable for thrombolytic therapy. Decreased chest pain, delay in seeking hospital admission, and nondiagnostic electrocardiographic findings contributed, in part, to the ineligibility of elderly patients. Hesitancy in treating this group is understandable because of the concern for co-morbid conditions that could increase the risk of complications, most significantly stroke. When does risk outweigh the benefits of thrombolytic therapy in older patients? Given the high mortality rate of elderly myocardial infarction patients and the fact that only a third of eligible elderly patients receive thrombolytic treatment, it may be time to reexamine our thrombolytic protocols. Before we do so, more needs to be known about the effectiveness of thrombolytic interventions in the older patient as well as who among the older population benefits the most with the least risk of complications.

Another subset of patients who are usually ineligible for the "silver bullet" are those who have received CPR. The reason for this is obvious—trauma and hemorrhage. However, the findings of Tenaglia et al. (Abstract 1–17) seriously challenge the practice of excluding all CPR patients from thrombolytic therapy. This retrospective study provides convincing evidence that CPR of less than 10 minutes' duration causes no added risk of hemorrhage. Although this study did not examine the effects of prolonged CPR, it does offer hope to many patients who require defibrillation and a short period of chest compression.

Nurses play a major role in identifying eligible patients for thrombolytic therapy. With further study, we will be able to take better aim when shooting our silver bullets, providing the greatest opportunity to those patients who can benefit the most. Maybe then we can afford to be smug.—C. Kessler, RN, MN, CCRN, CS

The Effect of Chronic Platelet Inhibition With Low-Dose Aspirin on Atherosclerotic Progression and Acute Thrombosis: Clinical Evidence From the Physicians' Health Study

Ridker PM, Manson JE, Buring JE, Goldhaber SZ, Hennekens CH (Brigham and Women's Hosp, Brookline, Mass)

Am Heart J 122:1588–1592, 1991 1–18

Problem.—Low-dose aspirin reduces the risks of cardiovascular disease, whether by reducing the risk of complete coronary occlusion at the time of thrombus formation or by decreasing atherosclerotic progression. Reduction of atherosclerosis should reduce rates of angina pecto-

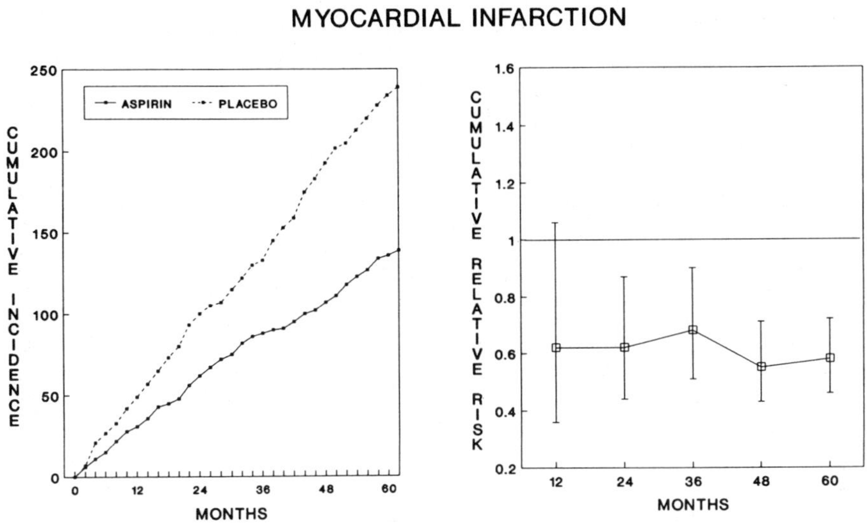

Fig 1–6.—Cumulative incidence and cumulative relative risk of first myocardial infarction among subjects randomized in the Physicians' Health Study, by month of follow-up. (Courtesy of Ridker PM, Manson JE, Buring JE, et al: *Am Heart J* 122:1588–1592, 1991.)

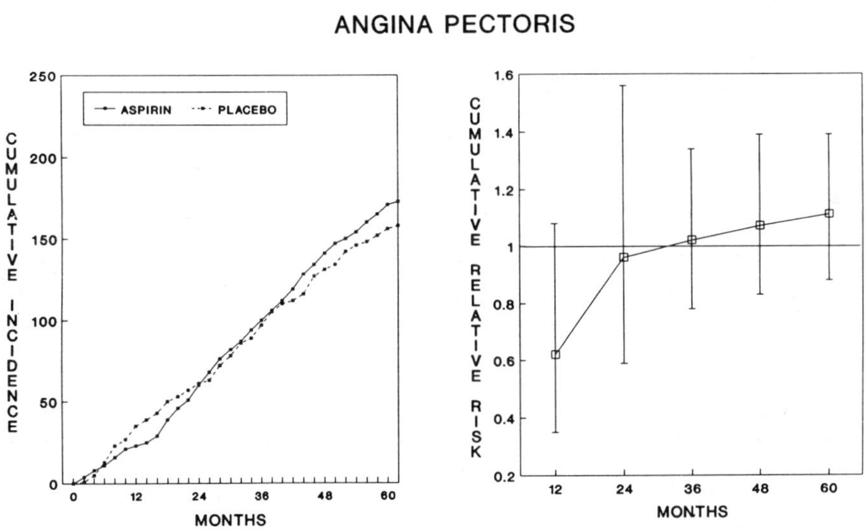

Fig 1–7.—Cumulative incidence and cumulative relative risk of having new angina pectoris among randomly assigned subjects in the Physicians' Health Study, by month of follow-up. (Courtesy of Ridker PM, Manson JE, Buring JE, et al: *Am Heart J* 122:1588–1592, 1991.)

ris. Data from The Physician's Health Study were used to describe the development of acute myocardial infarction and new angina pectoris among men randomly allocated to receive low-dose aspirin or placebo. The mechanisms by which long-term aspirin therapy reduced the risk of future coronary ischemia were also studied.

Study Methods.—The Physician's Health Study included 22,071 male physicians without previous myocardial infarction, transient ischemic attacks, or stroke. The subjects were randomly assigned to receive 325 mg of aspirin or a placebo every other day. At randomization, the mean age was 53.2 years in both groups. The men were treated and followed up for 5 years for the end points of myocardial infarction and new angina pectoris.

Findings.—The full protective effect of aspirin against myocardial infarction became apparent soon after the beginning of therapy and did not change significantly over time (Fig 1–6). Aspirin reduced the risk of first myocardial infarction by 44%. On the other hand, aspirin did not appear to reduce the risk of developing new angina pectoris at any time during the 5-year study period (Fig 1–7).

Conclusions.—Clinical data suggest that prophylactic low-dose aspirin inhibits acute thrombosis but does not slow the initiation and progression of atherosclerosis. Platelets may play a different role in acute thrombus formation than they do in the development of atherosclerotic plaque. Possible effects on development of atherosclerosis could be subclinical, but this would have to be investigated by quantitative angiography.

Comments: The Physician's Health Study has been heralded as a milestone in the continuing struggle against myocardial infarction (MI) (1). In fact, the results were so impressive that the study was prematurely terminated by an independent board monitoring the data. All participants were then notified immediately that the total number of MIs among subjects taking alternate day aspirin (325 mg) was reduced almost by half (1,2). The study was stopped because it would have been unethical to deny the benefits of these findings to the control group.

Results of a related international study found that aspirin therapy started within hours of acute MI reduced mortality by 23% (3). Recently, doses as low as 75 mg per day (4) have been found to be effective in reducing the risk of future cardiovascular events. In the current study by Ridker and colleagues, the mechanism responsible for MI risk reduction with low-dose aspirin therapy was evaluated. The data reveal that long-term platelet inhibition with alternate-day aspirin inhibits platelets during the critical period of plaque rupture but does not inhibit the progression of atherosclerosis, as demonstrated by reduced rates of new angina pectoris.

The results of these studies have important implications for us (5). Because chronic low-dose aspirin therapy reduces the risk of acute MI among healthy individuals and in patients with a history of MI, stroke, or unstable angina, we will encounter an increasingly greater number of patients receiving this prophylactic form of therapy. Thus, all patients admitted to our critical care units must be assessed carefully for chronic use of aspirin, especially those admitted for surgical or invasive procedures and those who may be suffering complications of such therapy (e.g., cerebral hemorrhage).

Teaching new patients about chronic aspirin therapy also is imperative. First, we must assess these patients for contraindications to aspirin (e.g., those at risk for hemorrhagic strokes or hemorrhagic complications such as peptic ulcer disease). These patients will need to understand that, although aspirin is beneficial in reducing the risk of acute MI, it does not reduce the progression of coronary artery disease. Thus, teaching related to coronary artery disease risk factor reduction is still essential.

When teaching these patients about aspirin, advise them to take the medication with milk, snacks, meals, or large volumes of water to help lessen gastric irritation. Inform them when and how often to take the medication. Emphasize the side effects of aspirin. Chronic therapy may increase excretion of vitamin C and decrease blood levels of folic acid; patients should probably be advised to take supplemental vitamin therapy (5). Instruct them to avoid the use of alcohol while on chronic aspirin therapy because both are irritating to the gastric mucosa. In some patients, this combination may increase the risk of gastrointestinal bleeding. Teach patients to observe for gastric irritation, stomach pain, heartburn, nausea and vomiting, and hypersensitivity reactions. They also need to monitor for unexplained bleeding or bruising, bleeding during toothbrushing or shaving, epistaxis, hematuria, and hemorrhoidal or gastrointestinal bleeding.

Aspirin is widely used for self-medication. Advise patients to read all drug product labels carefully because many cold remedies and other products contain aspirin. Teach patients to avoid combination products that contain aspirin. Because trade names may be confusing, instruct patients to read the list of ingredients carefully and check for the amount of aspirin in each dose, especially when comparing products with names like "arthritis strength" or "extra strength". Buffered formulations help to prevent gastric irritation, while enteric coated aspirin is designed to resist disintegration in the stomach by dissolving in the more neutral-to-alkaline environment of the duodenum, thereby preventing injury to the stomach. It is likely that many adverse effects of chronic aspirin therapy can be avoided by careful use and appropriate monitoring of the drug.—C.E. Guzzetta, RN, PhD, FAAN

References

1. Relman AS: Aspirin for the primary prevention of myocardial infarction. *N Engl J Med* 318:245–246, 1988.
2. The Steering Committee of the Physician's Health Study Research Group. Preliminary report: Findings from the aspirin component of the ongoing Physician's Health Study. *N Engl J Med* 318:262–264, 1988.
3. ISIS-2 Collaborative Group: Randomized trial of IV streptokinase, oral aspirin, both, or neither among 17,187 cases of suspected acute myocardial infarction. *Lancet* 2:340–360, 1988.
4. Wallentin and the Research Group on Instability in Coronary Artery Disease in

Southeast Sweden: Aspirin (75 mg/day) after an episode of unstable coronary artery disease: Long-term effects on the risk for myocardial infarction, occurrence of severe angina and the need for revascularization. *J Am Coll Cardiol* 18:1587–1593, 1991.

5. Karb VB: Selected cardiovascular drugs, in Guzzetta CE, Dossey BM (eds): *Cardiovascular Nursing: Holistic Practice*, St. Louis, Mosby–Year Book, 1992.

Effect of Monitoring Drug Concentrations Through Lines Used to Administer the Drugs: An In Vitro Study

Wanwimolruk S, Murphy JE (Univ of Otago, Dunedin, New Zealand; Mercer Univ, Atlanta, Ga)

Ther Drug Monit 13:443–447, 1991 1–19

Problem.—Drugs are given by intravenous catheters with increasing frequency, especially in critical care patients. It is tempting to withdraw blood samples for drug concentrations back through the catheter used to administer the drug to spare patients the discomfort of venipuncture, but this could result in false readings of monitored drug concentrations. An in vitro study was made of 3 different drugs and their potential to give falsely elevated concentrations when samples are withdrawn from the same line through which the medications are given.

Study Methods.—The drugs studied were digoxin, aminophylline, and phenytoin, given through central catheters in concentrations similar to those given clinically. The drug solutions were left in the catheter lumen for a duration similar to what occurs clinically. The solutions then either remained in the lumen or were flushed out with 5 mL of normal saline (NS). Six hours later, a sample was withdrawn for drug concentration analysis; in half of the lines, 5 mL of NS was drawn and discarded to simulate methods used to prevent contamination.

Findings.—With diluted drug administrations, minor artifactual drug concentrations were seen unless the line was flushed after drug administration or sample fluid was discarded before final sampling. With undiluted drug administrations, artifactual drug concentrations could only be prevented by flushing after the dose and discarding a sample before final sampling. It was also important, in some instances, to discard the syringe used to collect the discarded sample before collecting the final sample.

Conclusions.—Artifactual elevations of drug concentrations can occur when samples are withdrawn through the lines used to administer the drugs. In patients receiving undiluted drug concentrations, the catheter should be flushed just after the dose is given and a portion of the blood discarded before the final sample is taken. In patients receiving diluted drug concentrations, flushing after the dose or discarding a blood sample before final sampling is recommended.

Comments: This study provides validation for the common practice of blood sampling from indwelling catheters. We can now say, based on science and not merely on ritual, that flushing and discarding are the necessary methods to produce accurate blood sampling of drug concentrations. In fact, these researchers (both teaching in departments of pharmacy) noted *nursing* anecdotes as reasons for performing this study—too bad nurses didn't do it first! But this study can stimulate us to explore and validate this phenomenon further. That changes in medical treatment are based on drug concentration results makes this study important to replicate and then translate into practice. We need to know about other drugs—for example, antibiotics—and whether their response is the same. It also would be helpful to perform this study on actual patients to provide stronger validation and generalization of the findings.

The authors made an interesting point about the results with diluted versus undiluted drug concentrations. When no flushing or discarding was done with undiluted samples, the results were quite obviously artifactually altered. However, when no flushing or discarding was done with diluted samples, artifactual results were more subtle and therefore raise the concern that errors may be overlooked more easily.

This is a study of one of the "routines" of nursing that provides a scientific basis for practice. We need more.—S. Wingate, RN, DNSc, CCRN, CS

Defining the Proper Role for Self-Administered Sublingual Nitroglycerin: A Survey of Physicians and Patients
Bassan M (Kaiser Found Hosp, Bellflower, Calif)
Chest 100:34–38, 1991 1–20

Problem.—Patients with coronary artery disease, or suspected disease, are commonly prescribed sublingual nitroglycerin for self-administration. Over one 6-month period, 6 patients with adverse effects of this medication were seen. This prompted a survey of physicians and patients about the use of sublingual nitroglycerin.

Study Methods.—The survey included 112 cardiology outpatients who had myocardial infarctions. Eighty-six percent of the group were men with a mean age of 64 years and a mean of 8 years since their infarction. Also surveyed were 121 cardiologists and internists. Both questionnaires addressed the use of and opinions about sublingual nitroglycerin.

Findings.—Eighty-four percent of the physicians routinely prescribed nitroglycerin for their patients who had had a myocardial infarction, even for those without recurrent angina. A similar percentage of patients reported they kept their tablets with them at all times. In most cases, the patients used the tablets less than once a month, and many of the patients who always carried their medication with them had not used it once in the previous year. The majority of patients said they knew how to use the drug, but more than half said they would use it for dizziness, rapid heartbeat, or syncope. The patients reported it relieved their symptoms at least partially, although many of these symptoms would not likely be affected by nitroglycerin.

Conclusions.—Physicians should reexamine the practice of routinely prescribing nitroglycerin for patients who have had a myocardial infarction. It should be used for patients with well-defined, chronic angina during exertion or even recurrent angina at rest. Much of the claimed effectiveness of this drug appears to result from a placebo effect. It is often given to provide a sense of security.

Comments: It was surprising that this article was written by a physician, because the nursing implications of this study are powerful. The author concludes that physicians should reexamine their prescribing practices for sublingual nitroglycerin. However, no mention is made of how or whether these patients were taught to take their nitroglycerin—a nursing domain of practice. It sounds as if proper teaching would have prevented many of the untoward outcomes listed as the impetus for the author to perform the survey. Another issue not discussed by the author and related to patient education is that patients were surveyed an average of 8 years after myocardial infarction. One wonders whether patients even *remember* what they may (or may not) have been taught that long ago. Further, if patients used the nitroglycerin infrequently, as was noted in this study, they also may have forgotten how to take it correctly.

This study raises the question of how we teach the patients in the acute care setting. Patients seem to hear the parts about carrying nitroglycerin with them and how to take it. But they either don't remember, don't understand, or weren't taught about what it means to take a nitroglycerin pill and why trends or patterns in its use are so very important. I agree that nitroglycerin can certainly have detrimental effects when taken incorrectly, but I believe that the benefits of properly administered nitroglycerin can outweigh the risks. I also agree that physicians should evaluate their prescribing practices. Hopefully, each patient is reviewed individually to determine whether sublingual nitroglycerin is the right choice for him or her.

I think this author has provided intriguing data to challenge us as nurses to pursue this phenomenon further. This study could be replicated in other populations and at an earlier timeframe postmyocardial infarction. Current patient medication teaching programs could add an outpatient follow-up component to evaluate patient outcomes. A fascinating qualitative study would be to look at the decision-making process that patients go through when deciding how or whether to take a sublingual nitroglycerin.—S. Wingate, RN, DNSc, CCRN, CS

Description of Indicator Development for a Percutaneous Transluminal Coronary Angioplasty Monitor

Fields WL, Thomason TR (Sharp Memorial Hosp, San Diego, Calif)
J Nurs Care Qual 6:6–19, 1991 1–21

Purpose.—Perhaps the most difficult part of the quality assurance (QA) process is development of outcome and process indicators. Indicators for monitoring and evaluating patients treated with percutaneous transluminal coronary angioplasty (PTCA) were developed at Sharp Memorial Hospital.

Study Methods.—Percutaneous transluminal coronary angioplasty was chosen for monitoring because of the large volume of patients treated at the institution and because of the potential for complications in this population. A QA study of PTCA was developed by a subcommittee consisting of the QA coordinator and QA chairpersons from the relevant nursing units. Areas chosen for monitoring and evaluation were patient knowledge of the procedure and discharge instructions and patient conditions of hemodynamic stability and hematoma formation. The development of outcome indicators, including thresholds, was a difficult process. After a pilot study was done, indicators were revised. Data were then collected on 70 patients using patient interviews and chart abstraction.

Findings.—Patients were knowledgeable about the indications for PTCA and about their postdischarge care; however, one fourth of patients did not remember how to care for the angioplasty site at home. Chart abstraction revealed a low incidence of bleeding, hematoma formation, and reocclusion. Medical and nursing management were considered to be of high quality, although there was room for improvement in nursing documentation.

Discussion.—The development of a successful QA program for PTCA was described, focusing on the development of indicators. This process facilitated comprehensive, intradisciplinary evaluations of outcome and care and identified areas for improvement.

Comments: Quality assurance/quality improvement (QA/QI) is an integral part of all critical care units. Often the most tedious part of QA/QI at the unit level is the selection and development of indicators that are pertinent to clinical practice. This article gives excellent step-by-step directions for the selection, development, and use of a monitor for patients undergoing PTCA.

Enough detail is provided that other critical care units could use this as a template to guide them in this process. Perhaps some critical care units already use this process, but this group deserves credit for publishing their work so that others may benefit from this sharing rather than having to "re-invent the wheel."

Besides QA/QI, another benefit of this article is the emphasis on teamwork and group process. All of the units that interacted with this patient population were involved with monitor development–intensive care, telemetry, cardiac rehabilitation, and the cardiac catheterization laboratory. The use of brainstorming, multivoting, and group assignments facilitated their work. The authors listed strengths and limitations of the process and gave helpful suggestions for future refinement. This exemplifies a practical evaluation of a high-volume patient population that resulted in very doable changes in practice–that is, refinement of certain aspects of patient education and increased interrater reliability for chart abstraction.—S. Wingate, RN, DNSc, CCRN, CS

Cardiogenic Shock After Acute Myocardial Infarction: Incidence and Mortality From a Community-Wide Perspective, 1975 to 1988

Goldberg RJ, Gore JM, Alpert JS, Osganian V, de Groot J, Bade J, Chen Z, Frid D, Dalen JE (Univ of Massachusetts, Worcester)

N Engl J Med 325:1117–1122, 1991 1–22

Problem.—Cardiogenic shock continues to occur after myocardial infarction despite improved management. The records of 4,762 patients admitted with acute myocardial infarction to 16 hospitals in Massachusetts during a 14-year period were reviewed. Cardiogenic shock was defined by a systolic blood pressure below 80 mm Hg in the absence of hypovolemia, associated with cyanosis, cold extremities, altered mental status, ongoing oliguria, or congestive heart failure.

Patients.—The incidence of cardiogenic shock during the review period was 7.5%. The complication developed on the first hospital day in 44% of those affected and within the first 3 days in two thirds of patients. Older patients, women, and patients with recurrent or Q-wave infarcts were more likely to develop cardiogenic shock (table). More patients with cardiogenic shock than without it received digoxin, lidocaine, and other antidysrhythmic agents.

Findings.—Hospital mortalities were 78% for patients with cardiogenic shock and 13.5% for the others (Fig 1–8). Short-term survival for patients in cardiogenic shock did not improve during the period under review. In addition, long-term survival was significantly compromised in survivors of cardiogenic shock.

Conclusion.—Neither the incidence nor the prognosis of cardiogenic shock after acute myocardial infarction has improved in recent years.

Comments: The news is in, and it's not good: patients are still developing and dying of cardiogenic shock at the rate that they were 14 years ago. I suppose that these results are not surprising given the fact that patients in cardiogenic shock have lost 40% or more of their myocardial mass. It is important to note that data collection for this study ended in 1988. The authors state that, in this study, the limited use of the newer interventions and treatments to reduce infarct size and improve coronary perfusion (i.e., thrombolytic therapy and percutaneous transluminal coronary angioplasty), may have contributed to a failure to observe improvements in the incidence and mortality rate of cardiogenic shock. Therefore, assuming that medical practice patterns have changed in the last 5 years to reflect an increased use of these newer interventions, it will be imperative that this study be updated beyond 1988.

Characteristics of Patients With Acute Myocardial Infarction According to the Occurrence of Cardiogenic Shock

CHARACTERISTIC	(N = 358)	(N = 4404)	P VALUE*
	years		
Mean age	71.4	66.5	<0.001
	percent of group		
Male sex	51.4	62.2	<0.001
History			
Angina	27.1	26.8	NS
Diabetes	26.5	22.9	NS
Hypertension	42.5	47.0	NS
Myocardial infarction			
Initial episode	57.5	66.8	<0.001
Q wave	69.8	56.8	<0.001
Anterior location	50.6	48.9	NS
Peak creatine kinase ≥5 times normal	67.0	49.7	<0.001
Clinical complications			
Congestive heart failure	74.9	39.7	<0.001
Ventricular tachycardia	39.9	16.7	<0.001
Ventricular fibrillation	24.3	7.1	<0.001
Complete atrioventricular block	18.2	4.8	<0.001
Drug therapy			
Anticoagulants	58.9	66.0	<0.01
Antiplatelet agents	13.7	22.7	<0.001
Beta-blockers	19.3	41.5	<0.001
Calcium-channel blockers†	39.8	63.2	<0.001
Digoxin	53.1	35.8	<0.001
Lidocaine	59.5	43.0	<0.001
Other antiarrhythmic agents	34.6	22.6	<0.001
Nitrates	70.7	80.9	<0.001
Thrombolytic treatment†	7.6	15.0	<0.05
Diagnostic and interventional procedures			
Cardiac catheterization	7.8	10.5	NS
Coronary-artery bypass surgery	1.1	0.9	NS
Intraaortic balloon counter-pulsation	7.5	1.0	<0.001
Percutaneous transluminal coronary angioplasty†	1.7	2.5	NS
Pulmonary-artery catheterization	56.4	11.9	<0.001

* NS denotes a value that is not significant.
† Data were available for 1986 and 1988 only.
(Courtesy of Goldberg RJ, Gore JM, Alpert JS, et al: *N Engl J Med* 325:1117–1122, 1991.)

It is crucial to note that of the patients who develop cardiogenic shock, 44% of them do so within the first day after hospital admission. If these patients are to have a chance of survival, they must be treated rapidly and aggressively. The nursing implications here are clear. We need to maintain a high index of suspicion for all patients admitted to the coronary care unit with the presumptive diagnosis of acute myocardial infarction, especially during the first day of admission, to assess the clinical manifestations of car-

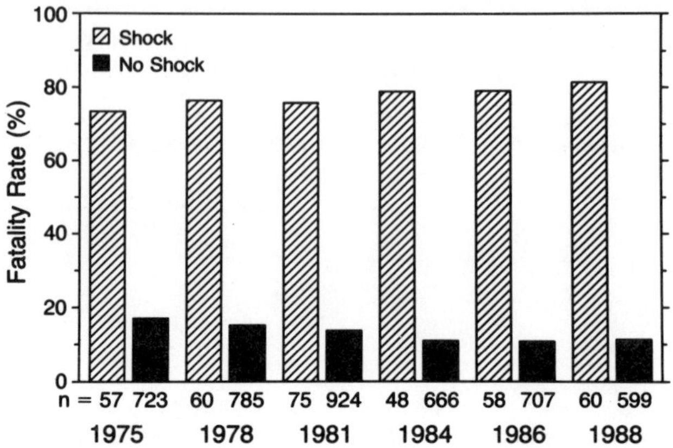

Fig 1–8.—In-hospital fatality rates among patients with acute myocardial infarction according to the year studied and the occurrence of cardiogenic shock. (Courtesy of Goldberg RJ, Gore, JM, Alpert JS, et al: *N Engl J Med* 325:1117–1122, 1991.)

diogenic shock. Essential assessment criteria must be identified so that early signs and symptoms can be recognized promptly. These include initial reductions in blood pressure and mean arterial pressure, reduced cardiac index, and elevated pulmonary artery wedge pressures; increases in heart rate progressing to a rapid thready pulse; dysrhythmias; altered mentation including lassitude, agitation, restlessness, and mental confusion; pale, cold extremities and cool moist skin progressing to cyanosis; reduced urinary output in the absence of hypovolemia; physical weakness; and signs and symptoms of congestive heart failure.

It has been reported that the early signs and symptoms of cardiogenic shock are more frequently identified by experienced critical care nurses (1). If this is true, then we need to provide guided experiences for new critical care nurses to enhance their ability to recognize early signs and symptoms. The literature also suggests that effective communication between the nurse and the physician may reduce the incidence of cardiogenic shock (1). Moreover, patient outcomes may depend on the effectiveness of the nurse's communication skills in reporting early signs and symptoms to the physician as well as the nurse's ability to obtain the appropriate response from the physician (1). Thus, we need to focus on some advanced practice tactics and develop in-service classes that integrate effective communication skills with power strategies to enhance autonomy and nurse-physician collaborative relationships (2). Our efforts could provide the vital link in changing the outcomes for these patients.—C.E. Guzzetta, RN, PhD, FAAN

References

1. Pyles SH: Role of the critical care nurse in the early detection and prevention of cardiogenic shock: Discovery of the weak link. *Heart Lung* 12:428, 1983.
2. Riegel B, Dossey BM: Acute myocardial infarction. in Dossey BM, Guzzetta CE,

Kenner CV (eds): *Critical Care Nursing: Body-Mind-Spirit,* ed 3. Philadelphia, JB Lippincott, 1992.

Effects of Basin Baths, Tub Baths, and Showers on Cardiovascular Response in 51 Healthy Men and Women

Winslow EH, Smith J (Univ of Texas at Arlington School of Nursing; Humana Hosp, Montgomery, Ala)

Cardiovasc Nurs 27:25–30, 1991 1–23

Problem.—Because little is known about normal cardiovascular responses to common bathing procedures, 51 healthy persons, most of them nurses, physicians, and other health-care providers, took part in a study to evaluate how bathing affects blood pressure, heart rate, presence of dysrhythmias, and perceived exertion.

Study Methods.—The ECG was recorded continuously, and indirect blood pressures were monitored as subjects randomly took a tub bath (water temperature 96–98°F); a basin bath (102–110°F); and a shower (96–98°F) at intervals of at least 10 minutes. After each bath they rated their perceived exertion using the Borg Scale. Of the 51 subjects, 39 were men and 12 were women.

Findings.—Before- and after-bath pulse rates differed more in men than in women. Men had a higher mean heart rate during tub bathing. For all subjects, peak heart rates during the basin bath were lower than during the tub bath but the differences between bathing type were not

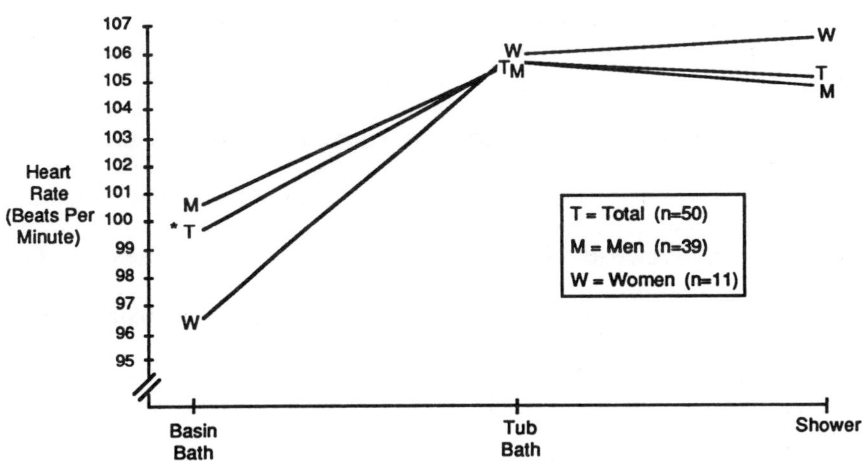

Fig 1–9.—Mean peak heart rate (beats/min) during basin bath, tub bath, and shower in 50 healthy subjects. (Courtesy of Winslow EH, Smith J: *Cardiovasc Nurs* 27:25–30, 1991.)

clinically dramatic (Fig 1-9). Four men had dysrhythmic responses. Post-bathing blood pressure was significantly higher in men than in women but were within normal ranges. Perceived exertion was similar after all baths, but subjects found the basin bath to be much less enjoyable than either the tub bath or shower. All forms of bathing took 5 to 6 minutes.

Conclusions.—It is not unusual for healthy adults to have a rise in pulse rate of 10 beats/minute or more after bathing in the hospital. Bathing carries an energy cost twofold to threefold above that of the resting level in healthy subjects. No marked differences in cardiovascular response were evident among tub bathing, basin bathing, and showering.

Comment: *See comment after Abstract 1–24.*

Shower Versus Sink Bath: Evaluation of Heart Rate, Blood Pressure, and Subjective Response of the Patient With Myocardial Infarction

Robichaud-Ekstrand S (Univ of Ottawa School of Nursing, Ottawa, Ontario)

Heart Lung 20:375–382, 1991 1–24

Problem.—An important issue in the early rehabilitation of patients who have myocardial infarction is how best to balance rest with physical activity to promote recovery most efficiently. This study compared the cardiovascular and subjective effects of a sitting shower with those of a sitting sink bath in low-risk myocardial infarction patients.

Study Methods.—Thirty patients who had had a myocardial infarction were monitored during the first 2 self-baths on consecutive days, 2 to 9 days after the event. In addition to monitoring the heart rate and blood pressure, ratings of perceived exertion (table) were acquired using the Borg Scale.

Findings.—All variables pointed to a significant effect of bathing, but recovery values of heart rate, blood pressure, and perceived exertion did not differ from resting values. Fatigue was the most common symptom both at rest and during bathing activities. Ten subjects had what was considered an atypical blood pressure or heart rate response to bathing. The 2 methods of bathing had comparable effects on the heart and on perceived exertion.

Nursing Implications.—A sitting shower is not more demanding than a sitting sink bath for low-risk myocardial infarction patients, allowing patients to select either of these options. It seems best, however, to replicate this study, taking care to record individual subjective responses carefully.

Comments: Any nurse who has taken care of patients who have had an acute myocardial infarction knows that they happily await permission to take their first hospital bath. The first study by Winslow and Smith (Abstract 1–23) points out the importance of studying normal responses of healthy persons

Borg Scale of Perceived Exertion, Symptoms, and Comments

Bath order	*1 (Sink—shower)* *2 (Shower—sink)*
1. Rate your exertion	Scores
7: Very very light	1
9: Very light	2
11: Fairly light	3
13: Somewhat hard	4
15: Hard	5
17: Very hard	6
19: Very very hard	7
2. Are you tired?	5—Yes 1—No
3. Are you short of breath?	5—Yes 1—No
4. Are you dizzy?	5—Yes 1—No
5. Do you have angina?	5—Yes 1—No
Overall subjective score (add 1 to 5)	
Comment section:	
6. Are you experiencing any other symptoms?	
7. Which bathing procedure did you prefer? 1—Sink 2—Shower	
8. What type of bath do you usually take at home? 1—Sink 2—Tub bath 3—Shower	

(Courtesy of Robichaud-Ekstrand S: *Heart Lung* 20:375-82, 1991.)

to bathing so that abnormal responses in sick persons can be recognized. Although this study revealed that there were no clinically dramatic differences among basin baths, tub baths, and showering in healthy subjects, it did raise important questions (and points out the need for further research) regarding gender differences that may exist in response to bathing, especially among sick persons. Another important finding was that pulse rate taken after bathing does not appear to be a good estimate of peak heart rate during bathing. Thus, the authors recommend that heart rates be monitored while the patient is bathing.

The second study by Robichaud-Ekstrand (Abstract 1–24) focuses on sick patients. The results of this study provide the scientific documentation to support the safe use of either a sitting sink bath or a sitting shower. It is interesting but not surprising to note that patients believed showering was easier and more enjoyable than a sink bath. Two previous studies also have been conducted to evaluate various types of bathing activities. Johnston et al. (1)

and Winslow (2) investigated the effects of shower, tub, and bed bathing on acute myocardial infarction patients. Johnston found that showering demanded greater oxygen consumption than either tub or bed bathing. Conversely, Winslow found that the physiologic cost of the 3 types of bathing were similar.

Although the findings from these studies were not identical, the study designs and the results provide us with important implications for bedside clinical practice. If patients are given a choice between a sitting shower or sitting sink bath, 2 to 9 days after their acute myocardial infarction, the following guidelines should be observed for safe practice:

- First, assess patients to be sure that they are at low risk for additional cardiac events (i.e., those without ongoing myocardial ischemia, severe left ventricular dysfunction, ventricular ectopy, or a resting heart rate greater than 90 beats/min. In addition, such low-risk patients should not have significant metabolic, thromboembolic, or musculoskeletal problems and should not be obese).
- Transfer patients to and from the bathing area by wheelchair.
- Provide a small stool for patients to sit on during the bathing period.
- Control the temperature of the sink or shower water between 35.5°C and 36.5°C (use a mercury-in-glass thermometer).
- Do not rush patients during the bathing period, but instruct them to limit bathing time to 5 minutes.
- Instruct patients to avoid washing their hair, back, and feet during the initial bathing period because of the additional energy expenditure involved.
- After bathing, assist patients with drying off and dressing to avoid additional and prolonged energy expenditure.

Because some of the low risk patients in Robichaud-Ekstrand's study did develop atypical cardiovascular responses and symptoms, it is still imperative that nurses assess the initial bathing responses of their patients. Heart rate, blood pressure, and the rate-pressure-product (heart rate × systolic blood pressure) should be evaluated before and after bathing. Heart rate should be monitored *during* bathing (telemetry units need to be waterproofed) to determine peak heart rate response. It is recommended that the Borg Scale with symptoms and comments (table) be used to evaluate the patient's subjective response.—C.E. Guzzetta, RN, PhD, FAAN

References

1. Johnston BL, Watt EW, Fletcher GF: Oxygen consumption and hemodynamic and electrocardiographic responses to bathing in recent post-myocardial infarction patients. *Heart Lung* 10:666–671, 1981.
2. Winslow EH: Oxygen uptake and cardiovascular responses in control subjects and acute myocardial infarction patients during bathing. *Nurs Res* 34:164–169, 1985.

Cardiopulmonary Resuscitation

Outcome After Cardiopulmonary Resuscitation in a Medical Intensive Care Unit

Peterson MW, Geist LJ, Schwartz DA, Konicek S, Moseley PL (Univ of Iowa, Iowa City)

Chest 100:168–174, 1991 1–25

Problem.—Cardiopulmonary resuscitation (CPR) is a commonly used procedure both in and out of the hospital. Its efficacy in modern critical care units, however, has not been studied. Such a study is important because patients in critical care units often have multisystem disorders and diseases reportedly associated with poor outcomes after CPR.

Study Methods.—The records of 114 patients who had CPR in 1 medical intensive care unit (MICU) during 3 years were reviewed to determine which clinical parameters influenced the outcome of CPR. The prearrest parameters evaluated were diagnoses, age, sex, duration of hospitalization, length of MICU stay, and severity of illness as measured by the acute physiology and chronic health evaluation (APACHE 2) scores. The arrest parameters evaluated were the initial cardiac rhythm and duration of CPR.

Demographics and Prearrest Clinical Characteristics of Subjects

Data	Group A	Group B	Group C
No. of subjects	80	21	13
Demographics			
Mean age, yr (range)	57 ± 18 (17-89)	56 ± 14 (28-80)	56 ± 11 (35-76)
Gender			
Male (%)	39 (49)	14 (67)	6 (46)
Female (%)	41 (51)	7 (33)	7 (54)
Prearrest clinical characteristics			
APACHE 2 score (range)	21.6 ± 8.8 (3-46)	18.3 ± 5.9 (4-28)	13.2 ± 5.6* (3-23)
Length of hospitalization prior to CPR, days (range)	10 ± 17 (1-100)	15 ± 20 (1-83)	15 ± 15 (1-44)
Length of ICU stay prior to CPR, days (range)	4 ± 11 (1-100)	6 ± 8 (1-32)	5 ± 6 (1-20)

* $P < .01$ compared with either group A or group B.

(Courtesy of Peterson MW, Geist LJ, Schwartz DA, et al: *Chest* 100:168–174, 1991.)

Findings.—Eighty patients, or 70%, were not resuscitated successfully. Twenty-one patients, or 18%, were resuscitated successfully but died later in the hospital. The median length of survival for this group was 3 days. Thirteen patients, or 11%, survived to hospital discharge. Only the prearrest parameters of hypotension and the Acute Physiology Score (APS) component of APACHE 2 differentiated those patients who survived until discharge from those who did not. Among arrest conditions, only the duration of resuscitative effort predicted the outcome of CPR (table). The average duration of CPR was almost 3 times as long in the nonsurviving groups as in the surviving group. Any patient who required more than 16 minutes of CPR did not survive to leave the hospital. There was no relationship between the other prearrest or arrest parameters (i.e., other diagnoses, age, sex, duration of hospitalization, length of MICU stay, and initial cardiac dysrhythmias) and the outcome after CPR.

Conclusions.—Cardiopulmonary resuscitation can be successful in patients in an MICU. Certain prearrest and arrest factors are useful in identifying patients most likely to benefit from CPR in critical care settings.

Comments: It is shocking to learn from the Peterson study that only 11% of the patients resuscitated in the MICU lived to be discharged from the hospital. It also is shocking to learn (from a related study by Gray) that of 185 patients presenting to an emergency department after an initially unsuccessful, but ongoing, resuscitation for a prehospital arrest, only 9% were resuscitated successfully in the emergency department and none survived to be discharged from the hospital (1).

It would be a monumental achievement to be able to predict who will and will not survive CPR for several reasons. Such predictions would provide physicians and nurses with clinical guidelines for identifying patients most likely to benefit from CPR. In addition, it could eliminate resuscitative efforts that result in outcomes of chronic vegetative states in patients after CPR (up to 10% in some studies) (2). Likewise, these predictions could be used to develop standards for do not resuscitate policies based on objective criteria to preempt efforts at resuscitation in patients who would not benefit from the results. The ability to predict survival also would serve to reduce hospital costs. Even if patients survive the initial CPR event, many have a high risk of dying before they are discharged from the hospital. In the Peterson study, for example, of those patients who were resuscitated successfully in the MICU, 62% died before they were discharged from the hospital. Such patients consume enormous institutional and economic resources. For these patients, CPR simply delays death and prolongs the act of dying—and in such situations has been called the $100,000 funeral (3).

Studies such as the ones by Peterson et al. and Gray are being seen more frequently in the literature and are urgently needed. The purpose of these studies is to identify *objective criteria* that can be used to predict the outcomes of patient care—in this case, the outcome is discharge survival of patients after CPR. Unfortunately, we know that objective criteria either are not available or are not being used in important clinical decisions such as do not resuscitate orders. Zimmerman et al., for example, evaluated the rationale (i.e., the use of objective criteria) behind do not resuscitate orders and could find none based on the patient's age, previous health, diagnosis, or severity of illness (4).

Although the findings from the study by Peterson et al. demonstrate that objective criteria such as hypotension, duration of CPR, and the APS component of the APACHE 2 are useful predictors of CPR survival, only the APS is practical in predicting survival *prior* to the arrest (because hypotension usually precedes the arrest by only a brief period and because duration of CPR is not known ahead of time). In a related study by Lawrence, attempts were made to uncover other objective criteria to predict the probability of CPR success in hospitalized patients with various combinations of risk factors (5). A classification system then was constructed to predict an individual's outcome based on these preexisting variables (e.g., shock, BUN > 20 mg/dL, Pao_2 < 60 mm Hg, and oliguria). Although the researchers were able to develop a model that accurately predicted survival percentage in a population of patients, the ability to predict CPR survival for an *individual patient* remained poor. A large percentage of cases in which patients actually survived would have been predicted to be failures based on their model. The authors concluded that preexisting variables do not accurately predict survival after CPR. Thus, it appears that we need more research to learn about additional variables and combinations of variables that predict CPR survivability before we can make sound predictions.

Nevertheless, there has been great emphasis lately on patients being involved in making treatment decisions. The Patient Self-Determination Act, the support of a durable power of attorney for health affairs, and the living will undoubtedly will have an impact on future decisions about initiating CPR or writing do not resuscitate orders. The research findings on predicting CPR survival will help to differentiate patients for whom CPR will offer benefit from those in whom CPR is futile. It also will assist physicians, nurses, and families in making these difficult decisions.—C.E. Guzzetta, RN, PhD, FAAN

References

1. Gray WA, Capone RJ, Most AS: Unsuccessful emergency medical resuscitation–Are continued efforts in the emergency department justified? *N Engl J Med* 325: 1393–1398, 1991.
2. Von Gunten DF: CPR in hospitalized patients: When is it futile? *Am Family Physician* 44: 2130–2134, 1991.
3. Schiedermayer DL, Shapiro RS: The conversational imperative: Discussing CPR with patients. *Med Ethics* 4: 6–10. 1989.
4. Zimmerman JE, Knaus WA, Sharpe SM, et al: The use and implication of do-not-resuscitate orders in the intensive care units. *JAMA* 255:351–356, 1986.
5. Lawrence ME, Price L, Riggs M: Inpatient cardiopulmonary resuscitation: Is survival prediction possible? *Southern Med J* 84:1462–1466, 1991.

Prevention of Oral Bacterial Flora Transmission by Using Mouth-to-Mask Ventilation During CPR

Cydulka RK, Connor PJ, Myers TF, Pavza G, Parker M (Case Western Reserve Univ, Cleveland, Ohio; Northwestern Memorial Hosp; Loyola Univ, Chicago)

J Emerg Med 9:317–321, 1991 1–26

Problem.—Bystanders are reluctant to perform mouth-to-mouth ventilation on people having cardiac arrest. This may have a significant impact on survival. The use of protective barrier precautions during cardiopulmonary resuscitation (CPR) has been recommended in areas in which the need for resuscitation is predictable. Seventeen ventilation devices were assessed to determine the adequacy of barrier protection against oral aerobic flora transmission.

Study Methods.—Eight of the devices tested were face shields, 8 were mask devices, and 1 was neither. All the mask devices and only 3 face shield devices contained one-way valves (Fig 1–10). The devices that contained such a valve were hypothesized to offer better barrier protection against the transmission of oral aerobic bacterial flora than devices not containing such a valve. The valves allowed air in from the rescuer side but did not let air out from the victim's side. All devices were disinfected, placed tightly over the investigator's face while he or she exhaled forcibly for 60 seconds, and then cultured for oral aerobic bacterial flora on the rescuer's side.

Findings.—Of the 17 devices, 7 (41%) were found to be contaminated with oral aerobic bacterial flora. None of the mask devices were contaminated with oral aerobic bacterial flora, compared with 6 face shields (table).

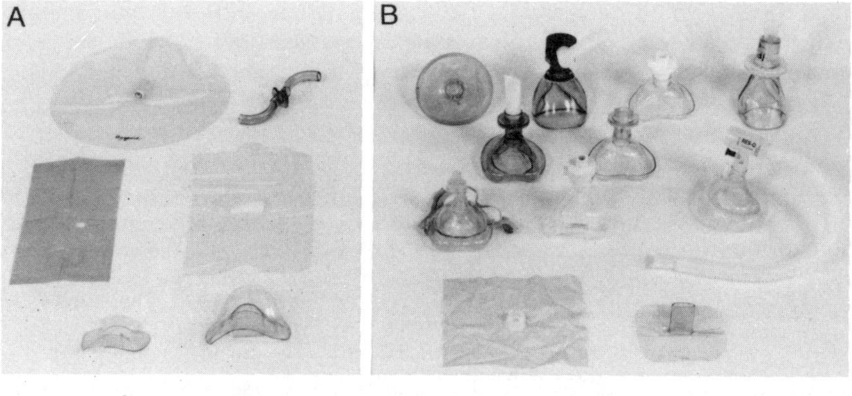

Fig 1–10.—A, devices lacking one-way valve: left to right: **top row:** Hygen-ic, Lifesaver; **second row:** Resusaid, Resusci; **bottom row:** MedCare, Samaritan. **B,** devices with one-way valves: left to right: **top row:** Sealeasy, Tru-fit, MTM Emergency Resuscitator, Res-Q-Flo, **second row:** Rightway Mouth-to-Mask Resuscitator, MTM Emergency Lung Ventilator; **third row:** Laerdal, Dyna Med, Res-Q-1; **bottom row:** Portex, CPR Microshield. (Courtesy of Cydulka RK, Connor PJ, Myers TF, et al: *J Emerg Med* 9:317–321, 1991.)

	Results of Culture	
	Positive Culture† (*n* = 20 trials)	Negative Culture‡ (*n* = 20 trials)
Faceshields*	Hygen-ic®†	CPR Microshield®‡
	MedCare Mask®†	Portex®‡
	Resusci®†	
	Resusaid®†	
	Samaritan®†	
	Sealeasy®†	
Mask devices*		Laerdal®‡
		Dyna Med®‡
		MTM Emergency Lung Ventilator®‡
		MTM Emergency Resuscitator®‡
		Res-Q-Flo®‡
		Res-Q-1®‡
		Rightway Mouth-to-Mask‡ Resuscitator®‡
		Trufit®‡
Tube devices	Lifesaver®†	

* $P < .007$ by Fisher's exact test.
† Each device tested had a positive culture in 20 of 20 trials.
‡ Each device tested had a negative culture in 20 of 20 trials.
(Courtesy of Cydulka RK, Connor PJ, Myers TF, et al: *J Emerg Med* 9:317–321, 1991.)

Conclusions.—All ventilation devices with a one-way valve, except the Sealeasy device, had adequate barrier-type protection from oral aerobic bacterial flow during mouth-to-mouth ventilation simulation and are recommended for use. These conclusions are limited because the transmission of anaerobic oral bacterial flora or viruses was not tested and because barrier protection was tested for only 60 seconds, not over the normal course of CPR. Victim barrier protection from an infected rescuer also needs to be addressed in future research.

Comments: The fear of disease transmission during mouth-to-mouth ventilation is legitimate, given the array of viral and bacterial illnesses that can be spread through respiratory droplets or by contact with infected saliva (e.g., rubella, tuberculosis, meningococcal infections). Hepatitis B can be acquired when infected blood or saliva contact lesions in the oral mucosa (1). Likewise, HIV has been isolated from the saliva (2). Although it has not been determined that HIV can be transmitted by saliva, the situation is disquieting to health care workers and to the general public. As a result, CPR practices have been impacted. For example, it is known that the pool of CPR trainees has declined over recent years and that first responders to the scene of a cardiac arrest have refused to perform mouth-to-mouth ventilation (3). To address these concerns, it is predicted that the American Heart Association will mandate that health professionals learn how to perform mouth-to-mask breathing in their basic life support courses. It also is expected that laypersons will be taught mouth-to-mouth ventilation using a simpler protective device such as a face shield (4).

There are at least 30 oropharyngeal devices currently on the market. The question is, which ones are best? The study by Cydulka and colleagues revealed that face shields were useless in preventing transmission of oral bacterial unless they contained a one-way valve. (However, one face shield, Sealeasy, which did contain a one-way valve, was consistently contaminated with bacteria, and the authors could not explain why). On the other hand, all of the face masks with one-way valves were effective in preventing transmission of bacteria (see table). Thus, it appears that one-way valves make a difference—at least in the transmission of bacteria.

What other objective criteria should be used to determine which devices are best? It is suggested that face shields and facemasks be evaluated for ventilatory efficiency, ease of use, cost, and convenience in terms of portability. One new device, a one-piece silicone mask called the Kiss of Life [KOL] has been found to meet this criteria (3) (i.e., excellent ventilatory characteristics, easy to use, disposable, can be carried in the pocket, and experimentally impermeable to HIV, although transmission of other viruses and bacterial flora were not evaluated).

As nurses who perform CPR and teach others to do so, we have the responsibility of choosing the best device currently available—the best for ourselves, those we teach, and for our patients. This is a hot topic not only because of the impetus to prevent disease transmission but also because of the finances involved (i.e., fiscal gains to the manufactures and additional costs passed to hospitals, health care providers, and CPR students). I suspect we will see many more comparative studies that evaluate the advantages and disadvantages of various airway devices in the future, and thus, it will be critical that we stay abreast of this literature.—C.E. Guzzetta, RN, PhD, FAAN

References

1. Powell EK, Duke M, Cooksley WGE: Hepatitis B transmission within families: potential importance of saliva as a vehicle of spread. *Aust NZ J Med* 15:717–720, 1985.
2. Friedland GH, Klein RS: Transmission of the human immunodeficiency virus. N *Engl J Med* 1125–1135, 1987.
3. Lightsey DM, Shah PK, Forrester JS, et al: A human immunodeficiency virus-resistant airway for cardiopulmonary resuscitation. *Am J Emerg Med* 10:73–77, 1992.
4. Willens JS: BCLS forecast: Big changes in the wind. *Nurs '91* November:53–56, 1991.

Potential for Injury: Trauma After Cardiopulmonary Resuscitation

Sommers MS (Univ of Cincinnati, Ohio)

Heart Lung 20:287–295, 1991 1–27

Questions for Future Research

1. Which types of hospital in-service CPR training best limit CPR injuries? Should CPR training differ for ICU versus ward nurses?
2. At what point in the resuscitation are rib and sternal fractures most likely to occur: early in the resuscitation or late?
3. What is the optimum time for each resuscitator to provide compressions? Is there a relationship between the length of time one resuscitator provides chest compressions and CPR injury?
4. Is there a relationship between hand size of the resuscitator providing chest compressions and the incidence of rib and sternal fractures?
5. Which type of backboard or adjuncts to CPR best limit vertebral injury during chest compressions in geriatric victims with osteopenia or kyphosis?
6. Are there relationships between incidence of CPR injury and age, sex, and body surface area of victims?
7. Is there a relationship between type of conductant material used for defibrillation and injury to the skin after defibrillation?
8. Which intervention best limits gastric distension and rupture during CPR: nasogastric intubation and suction or needle decompression through the anterior abdominal wall?
9. Which adaptations in resuscitator bags would decrease the incidence of pulmonary barotrauma with CPR?
10. Are female victims more likely to be injured during CPR than male victims?

(Courtesy of Sommers MV: *Heart Lung* 20:287–295, 1991.)

Problem.—Cardiopulmonary resuscitation (CPR) is a lifesaving technique that almost all critical care nurses and physicians perform. However, CPR has the potential to cause serious injury. Practitioners who are informed about these injuries and ways to avoid them can reduce the incidence of injury.

Incidence.—Various autopsy series report an overall CPR complication rate of 21% to 65%. A study of CPR survivors disclosed a noncardiac complication rate of 35%. Incidence of injury is affected by the location of the arrest and the patient's diagnosis. The rate is lower in the intensive care unit and higher on the ward and in patients with pneumonia.

Classification.—Most CPR-related injuries affect the skin or thorax; others may involve the upper airway, abdomen, lungs, heart, and great vessels. Skin injuries, such as chest abrasions, external chest contusions, and defibrillator burns are easily assessed by inspection. Thoracic injuries include rib and sternal fractures, flail chest, mediastinal hemorrhage, pneumothorax and hemothorax, and rib contusion. In autopsy series, 19% to 52% of subjects have at least 1 broken rib. Airway injuries can include the presence of upper airway vomitus as well as intubation injuries. Injury from improperly placed stylets is considered avoidable. Many cases of pneumonia in CPR survivors result from aspiration of stomach contents. This complication is assessed by monitoring for fever, hypoxemia, and dyspnea, evaluating pulmonary secretions, and auscultating for wheezes and crackles. Abdominal injuries may include esophageal and gastric rupture, often related to the esophageal obturator airway, and liver injury, including puncture by a broken rib. Pulmonary barotrauma is sometimes observed. The heart and great vessels may be injured by chest compression, central line placement, or intracardiac injection of medications. A variety of miscellaneous injuries has also been reported.

Discussion.—The incidence of injuries related to the trauma of CPR can be minimized by careful attention to proper CPR techniques. Questions that are appropriate for future research are listed in the table.

Comments: This article would be particularly suited as the basis for an inservice discussion on preventing CPR-related injury. It is thorough, up to date, and includes the current statistics on the incidence of injuries classified according to anatomical location. In addition, the author skillfully details specific signs and symptoms to be assessed in the postresuscitation period to detect CPR-related injury. This information could be used to develop a systematic postresuscitation assessment format for survivors of CPR.

I am frequently asked by nurses how they can get more involved in research. The research questions at the end of the article would be a good place to begin. They are particularly insightful (see table) and would lend themselves well to investigation by nurses. For example, research question 4 hypothesizes that there may be a relationship between the resuscitator's hand size and the development of sternal and rib fractures. Presumably, the larger the hand, the higher the incidence of fractures. Clinicians could easily carry out this study by developing a systematic method to measure various resuscitators' hand length and width and compare this information to clinical observations and chest x-rays that confirm the diagnosis of rib or sternal fractures in postresuscitation patients. Several other research questions listed in the table are straightforward and would be relatively easy to investigate.

In addition to the research questions posed in the table, it is especially interesting to me that the data presented in this article indicate that patients resuscitated on the ward have a 32% incidence of complications while patients in the intensive care unit have only a 12% incidence. Why is there almost a threefold difference? Is it related to different CPR training between the ward and the intensive care unit, different motivation, or the "lose it if you don't use it" syndrome of performance skills? There are many questions that remain to be answered, and I urge my colleagues to consider this rich field of research.—C.E. Guzzetta, RN, PhD, FAAN

Preliminary Development of Two Predictive Models for DNR Patients in Intensive Care

Tittle MB, Moody L, Becker MP (Univ of South Florida, Tampa; Univ of Michigan, Ann Arbor)

Image: J Nurs Scholarship 23:140–144, 1991 1–28

Problem.—The most seriously ill patients in the intensive care unit (ICU) often have poor outcomes and use a large share of medical and nursing resources, especially ICU patients with do not resuscitate (DNR) orders. Variables that would best predict a DNR classification were identified and a model for predicting what nursing care would be required by DNR patients in the ICU was developed.

Study Methods.—Sixty-two patients with DNR orders and 62 without such orders in the ICUs of 3 community hospitals were compared. Nursing care requirements, severity of illness, resources allocation, and sociodemographic characteristics were analyzed (table).

Findings.—The best predictors of DNR classification were origin of admission and severity of illness score on the day of admission to the ICU. The best predictors of nursing care requirements for ICU patients with the DNR classification were number of days spent in intensive care before the DNR order, the average daily resource allocation points after the DNR order, and the severity of illness score on the day the DNR order was given.

Conclusions.—In the ICU, patients classified as DNR still need laborintensive nursing care and treatments, even though the DNR order implies that the patient is hopelessly ill. Clearly, DNR orders do not suggest abandoning the patient. Do not resuscitate decisions and treatment decisions must be separate, although discussions with the patient and

Sociodemographic Characteristics of Sample

	DNR Patients (n=62)	Non-DNR Patients (n=62)
Age (mean yr)	74	67.7
Residence (%)		
Nursing Home	21	8
Home/Family	79	92
Ethnic Group (%)		
White	97	84
Non-white	3	16
Gender (%)		
Male	47	53
Female	54	46
Martial Status (%)		
Married	42	58
Divorced	8	5
Widowed	36	25
Separated	2	0
Single	8	13

(Courtesy of Tittle MB, Moody L, Becker MP: *Image: J Nurs Scholarship* 23:140–144, 1991.)

family should include whether certain treatments will be beneficial or only prolong death unnecessarily.

Comments: Should patients with a do not resuscitate (DNR) status be admitted to an intensive care unit (ICU)? Should they remain in the ICU once the DNR order is written? According to groups like the American Thoracic Society, the answer is yes, if there is hope that life-sustaining therapy can achieve a meaningful survival for the patient (1). Do not resuscitate orders are independent of treatment decisions and therefore do not preclude other medical and nursing interventions. Thus, a DNR order is *not* a part of a broader order that includes "care and comfort" only.

A growing number of patients are being admitted to the ICU with DNR orders. Serious questions have been raised regarding whether such admissions are warranted given the increased nursing and medical resources used for such patients and the high cost of ICU stays. In 1 study, 14% of the 506 patients admitted to the ICU were designated as DNR (2). Because such patients continue to receive aggressive therapy, their nursing care needs remain high.

The study by Tittle et al. adds to the growing body of knowledge aimed at predicting the outcomes of illness and illness-related situations. These predictions then are used to guide physicians and nurses in making decisions regarding treatment options as well as in developing criteria for allocation of resources. The models proposed by the researchers give us additional data by which to discuss certain treatments with families and patients to decide whether they might have a possible benefit in terms of patient outcome and quality of life or whether they are needlessly prolonging death. Likewise the continued development of predictive models for nursing care will supply objective criteria for decisions regarding the nursing care requirements of DNR patients in ICU. It also will assist in allocation of nurses and resources needed to care for such patients. It must be remembered, however, that such predictive models remain an inexact science when applied to individual patients.

This article will be particularly useful for critical care nurses because it imparts a sound nursing perspective by which to evaluate and predict the nursing care needs of DNR patients. Based on the ethical principle of just allocation of scarce resources, however, I believe that it is important that we continue to evaluate whether care of the DNR patient is justified in the ICU.—C.E. Guzzetta, RN, PhD, FAAN

References

1. American Thoracic Society Bioethics Task Force: Withholding and withdrawing life-sustaining therapy. *Am Rev Respir Dis* 144:726–731, 1991.
2. Lewandowski W, Daly B, McClish DK, et al.: Treatment and care of "do not resuscitate" patients in a medical intensive care unit. *Heart Lung* 14:175–181, 1985.

Others

Effects of Timing and Reinforcement of Preoperative Education on Knowledge and Recovery of Patients Having Coronary Artery Bypass Graft Surgery

Cupples SA (Potomac, Md)
Heart Lung 20:654–660, 1991 1–29

Problem.—Although patients benefit from preoperative educational interventions, fiscal constraints in the 1980s have severely limited the amount of time available for such interventions. Patients are now admitted the day before surgery, and preoperative education is relegated to that afternoon or evening. Unfortunately, patient anxiety over the impending surgery increases as the day approaches, and high anxiety levels impede learning. The efficacy of preadmission preoperative education for patients undergoing coronary artery bypass graft surgery (CABG) was investigated.

Independent t Tests for Outcome Measures

Variable	*Mean*	*SD*	DF	t	p
KQ scores					
Experimental group	18.74	1.34	38	3.87	<0.001
Control group	16.85	1.66			
STAI scores					
Experimental group	32.80	7.91	38	1.20	0.24
Control group	36.96	13.27			
POMS TMD scores					
Experimental group	10.40	20.69	38	2.31	0.03
Control group	36.00	45.09			

Abbreviations: KQ, Coronary Artery Bypass Graft Surgery Knowledge Questionnaire; *STAI,* State-Trait Anxiety Inventory; *POMS TMD,* Profile of Mood States total mood disturbance.

(Courtesy of Cupples SA: *Heart Lung* 20:654–660, 1991.)

Study Methods.—Forty patients scheduled for an initial elective CABG procedure were enrolled in the randomized, experimental, posttest-only study. Patients in the experimental group received preoperative education 5–14 days before admission and a follow-up phone call 4 days before admission in addition to the routine postadmission preoperative education, whereas patients in the control group received only the routine postadmission preoperative intervention. Outcome measures included preoperative knowledge of CABG surgery (measured by a CABG surgery knowledge questionnaire) and routine postoperative state anxiety (State-Trait Anxiety Inventory), postoperative mood state (profile of mood status), and physiologic recovery (Woffer-Davis Recovery Inventory).

Findings.—State anxiety levels of patients were significantly lower 5–14 days before the procedure than on the night before surgery. Patients who received both preadmission and postadmission preoperative education had significantly higher levels of knowledge before the surgery, more positive postoperative mood states, and more favorable physiologic recoveries than patients receiving only postadmission preoperative education (table).

Conclusions and Nursing Implications.—Patients in the experimental group and their families responded positively to the preadmission teaching session and a follow-up telephone call. Patients in the experimental group probably learned more because their initial educational session occurred when they were less anxious. Patients in the control group received their educational intervention the day before surgery, a time when they were more likely to be anxious.

Comments: This study substantiates a notion that most of us intuitively already know—that the day before surgery is a stressful time for most preoperative CABG patients. It also confirms a well established fact—that high levels of stress interfere with learning. Based on the knowledge gained from both intuition and science, we need to seriously question our traditional methods of patient education. Sandra Cupples has done part of this for us by unveiling the important issue of *timing* related to preoperative teaching. Although the sample size is small, and the study design may have some problems (like maybe the experimental group got more attention), the findings brought forth an "ah-hah" response from me. Can any of us really believe that preoperative teaching will be effective when presented the day before a major stressful surgical event? It is imperative that we acknowledge the findings from this study and the common sense it transmits.

We have long been told that the practice of nursing cannot be based on hunches (even if some of those hunches are good ones). Administrators want facts based on scientific documentation before changes in traditional, time-honored practices can occur, particularly when finances are involved. Thus, I would recommend that the effect of timing on preoperative education be replicated in the future on a variety of patient groups. My guess is that the results will be the same. Nonetheless, we would then have the facts and the data to support the need to change our patient education practices so that preoperative education would be provided before admission.

Because it was found that anxiety was low 5–14 days before surgery, this would appear to be the ideal time to initiate preoperative teaching. Preadmission preoperative teaching could be accomplished in the physician's office, clinic, on an outpatient basis, or during the time of preadmission laboratory testing instead of in the hospital the day before (or just hours before) surgery. If we could change our practice by teaching patients in nontraditional settings during the time period when they are not highly anxious, it is likely that they would understand and learn more, as Cupples has pointed out, related to *what* will be happening, *where* it will happen, *when* it will be happening, *why* it is happening, and most important, *how* they can best facilitate their own recovery. Patients might then have the opportunity to mentally walk through the experience and psychologically prepare for it. This is called the process of coping. This could have an enormous effect not only on learning but also on postoperative psychophysiologic recovery. Somehow this just seems like common sense.—C.E. Guzzetta, RN, PhD, FAAN

2 Respiratory Dysfunction

Guidelines for Standards of Care for Patients With Acute Respiratory Failure on Mechanical Ventilatory Support

Task Force on Guidelines of the Society of Critical Care Medicine

Crit Care Med 19:275–278, 1991 2–1

Purpose.—The Task Force on Guidelines of the Society of Critical Care Medicine has established minimum standards of care for patients with acute respiratory failure who are receiving mechanical ventilation in the critical care unit. Guidelines about personnel, monitoring, support services, equipment, general management, and ventilator management were outlined.

Guidelines.—Available personnel should include the primary or consultant physician, in-house personnel who can provide advanced cardiac life support and tracheal intubation, nurses at a minimum ratio of 1 to every 2 patients, and at least 1 respiratory therapist. Equipment for continuous monitoring of cardiac rate and rhythm, hemoglobin, end-tidal carbon dioxide, blood pressures, and core temperature should be available. Available support services should include radiography, laboratory services, and respiratory services. Assist control, intermittent mandatory pressure support, and controlled mechanical ventilation modalities are to be available. Guidelines for general management should address initial evaluation, vital signs, need for continuous and periodic monitoring, preventive measures, and available therapies or diagnostic modalities. For ventilator management, the physician should direct airway management, ventilatory support, and removal of ventilatory support as appropriate for the patient. Attention should be given to prevention of unplanned extubation, suctioning of secretions by sterile technique, and maintaining oxygen saturation at 90% or greater. The physician should consider the frequency of blood gas analysis and the measures that will be used to achieve patient comfort, including sedation and an arterial line. Weaning is to be based on objective observations and followed by observation.

Implications.—These minimum standards of care for patients with acute respiratory failure must be met by all critical care units. Many units will exceed most or all of the guidelines. When exceptions to the standards are unavoidable, the reasons must be documented.

Comments: This set of guidelines from the Society of Critical Care Medicine is an important recommendation on the management of patients with mechanical ventilatory support. The important points of the guidelines include recommended nursing and technologic support. The reason these points are important is to attempt to develop a minimum standard in the management of perhaps the most critically ill patients in the critical care unit setting. I believe all units should take note of these recommendations, particularly since they are not unreasonable. It is also likely, however, that many critical care units do not adhere to these guidelines. These units are at an increased risk of delivering less than optimal patient care and are also at an increased legal risk. As pointed out in the guidelines, if for any reason these guidelines cannot be met, the reasons should be documented. Considering mechanical ventilation management will increase in complexity and technologic support (e.g., continuous blood gases), these minimal standards are essential for any critical care unit.—T. Ahrens, RN, DNS, CCRN

Building a Critical Path for Ventilator Dependency

Thompson KS, Caddick K, Mathie J, Newlon B, Abraham T (Univ Hosp of Cleveland)

Am J Nurs 91:28–31, 1991 2–2

Problem.—More and more elderly patients are recovering from life-threatening events in traditional intensive care units (ICUs). A nursing case-management plan geared to these patients' specific problems is needed. Typically, these patients develop complications after cardiothoracic or vascular surgery and cannot be weaned from ventilation within 2 or 3 days. Because ventilator-dependent ICU patients are clinically stable, they are assigned a lower priority than hemodynamically unstable patients. Continuity of care for these ventilator-dependent patients can suffer, and costs can rise.

Critical Path.—A committee of case managers at 1 center collaborated with the medical director, nutritionist, social worker, and physical and occupational therapists to develop a critical path for ventilator-dependent patients. The committee considered the patients' multiple diagnostic-related-groups (DRGs) and their weaning, nutrition, and activity. The critical path is an abbreviated protocol for key incidents that must occur in a predictable or timely order to keep length of stay appropriate. It identifies key tasks or events as they relate to patient problems rather than to nursing or medical diagnoses. Discharge planning, ventilator dependency, fluid balance, nutrition, elimination, sleep pattern, and activity issues are included. Discharge or transfer is accomplished on day 29.

Conclusions.—This critical, or anticipated recovery, path for ventilator-dependent patients will be further refined as new subgroups with specific needs emerge.

Comments: The concept of critical paths spread with great speed throughout health care after their introduction from the business sector. This is interesting in light of the absence of any studies that support their specific value. Despite the lack of objective studies, the concept is worthy of investigation because of its potential impact on resource expenditures.

The authors of this article on the long-term mechanical ventilation critical path provide a good example of an inclusive guideline for care (see table). However, like all critical paths, excellent goals are usually provided, but the adherence to specific time frames limits credibility. This critical path illustrates the limits of time goals rather than of event goals. For example, the weaning plan states that the patient will be placed on a tracheotomy collar on day 22. This arbitrary designation may have been determined by the authors from their experience; however, no objective research exists to designate this day as the time that a tracheotomy collar would be used. Granted, the critical path does not limit the speed at which one can progress, but to give arbitrary times that do not have research support is little better than guessing.

For a critical path to have a consistent impact on patient outcome, we must do better than guess. Bear in mind, the authors of this article do a good job of identifying key factors that could have an impact on the outcome of a ventilator-dependent patient. However, the article also includes some of the concerns clinicians have when presented with concepts like critical paths. For critical paths to truly have an impact on resource expenditures, they must provide key elements that the clinician must consider in the care of the patient. They must not get bogged down with arbitrary time guidelines that limit their credibility to the clinician.—T. Ahrens, RN, DNS, CCRN

Control of Blood Gas Measurements in Intensive-Care Units

Roberts D, Ostryzniuk P, Loewen E, Shanks A, Wasyluk T, Pronger L, Hasinoff I, Roberts E, McEwen TAJ (University of Manitoba, Winnipeg)
Lancet 337:1580–1582, 1991 2–3

Problem.—Because blood gas measurements are the most common laboratory study in the intensive care unit (ICU), it is surprising that so little is known about appropriate indications for testing or optimal frequency. A prospective investigation monitored the frequency of blood gas measurements in 2 adult ICUs for 7 months before and 12 months after introducing a protocol of indications for testing.

Methods.—The appropriate use of pulse oximeters was encouraged. In most patients the lowest acceptable limit of arterial oxygen saturation was set at 90% or greater (Fig 2–1). There were 647 patients prospectively enrolled in the 7-month preprotocol phase and 1,236 patients en-

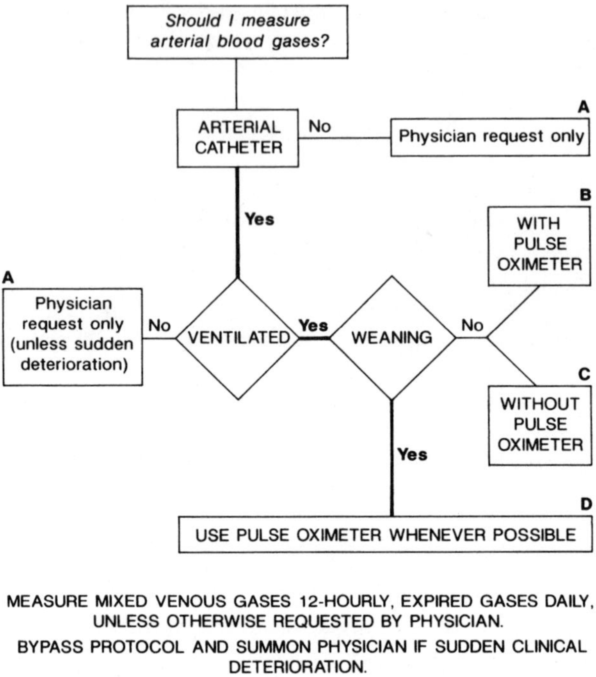

Fig 2–1.—Protocol for use of blood gas measurements. (Courtesy of Roberts D, Ostryzniuk P, Loewen E, et al: *Lancet* 337:1580–1582, 1991.)

rolled in the 12-month phase after the protocol was established. The 2 sets of patients were comparable demographically and with respect to acute physiology and chronic health evaluation scores and survival.

Findings.—The frequency of blood gas analysis declined 44% after introduction of the protocol. A nursing survey failed to reveal any adverse events that might have resulted from less frequent blood gas sampling. Those asked reported that the protocol encouraged clinical decision-making in line with their training and skills.

Nursing Implications.—A simple protocol can substantially limit the need for blood gas measurements in the ICU without undue morbidity resulting. No cases of severe unexpected hypoxia or hypercapnia occurred.

Comments: This is an interesting article continuing a trend in recent years citing the impact of implementing a multidisciplinary blood gas protocol in a critical care setting. The authors have compiled a large sample size to add value to the study. Whereas one might question some aspects of the protocol, such as its clarity, (Fig 2–1) and the use of oximetry values as low as 85% (because actual oxyhemoglobin values are usually several percentage points lower than pulse oximetry values), the focus of the study is what is important. The authors demonstrated no known alteration in quality of care despite a substantial (44%) reduction in blood gas usage. Economically, a tremendous savings was realized, although the exact numbers are difficult to compute. What this type of article points out is the need to use technology such as pulse oximeters to change practice. To continue using past practices when technology affords an opportunity for advancement is wasteful and inefficient. Development of protocols for the use of oximetry to replace blood gases (drawn only for Pa_{O_2} or Sa_{O_2} values) is a logical way to proceed in advancing nursing practice in this area. From articles such as this, it is becoming increasing clear that the collaboration between nursing, medicine, and other health professionals such as respiratory therapists is the appropriate way to proceed to improve quality of care while simultaneously reducing costs.—T. Ahrens, RN, DNS, CCRN

Sa_{O_2} Monitoring in the Postanesthesia Care Unit

Berels DJ, Marz MS (St Joseph Mercy Hosp, Pontiac, Mich)

J Post Anesth Nurs 6:394–401, 1991 — 2–4

Problem.—Postanesthesia monitoring has been greatly affected by the recent introduction of pulse oximetry. Reported postanesthesia care unit (PACU) impact events have decreased, possibly because of Sa_{O_2} monitoring. A pilot study was performed to determine objectively the patient's respiratory status on PACU discharge by using Sa_{O_2}, to assess the need for respiratory support based on Sa_{O_2}, to evaluate the relationship between temperature and Sa_{O_2}, and to collect baseline data on PACU use of pulse oximetry and supplemental oxygen.

Study Methods.—The investigators collected data on modified Aldrete scores (a postanesthetic evaluation scale) and Sa_{O_2} measurements before and after surgery, oxygen use, PACU time, and patient temperature. Fifty-six patients were studied, representing a convenience sample of patients undergoing cholecystectomy, hysterectomy, or bowel resection. Sa_{O_2} was measured by a pulse oximeter with a clip probe.

Findings.—Modified Aldrete scores and PACU discharge Sa_{O_2} values were moderately and inversely correlated—higher Aldrete scores of 8–10 were associated with lower Sa_{O_2} discharge values. This was not statistically significant, but the authors viewed it as clinically significant. There was a significant relationship between patient temperature and Sa_{O_2} values on room air. There was an inverse association between length of PACU stay and Sa_{O_2} values on room air—patients with Sa_{O_2} values of 85% to 90% stayed in the PACU for 3 hours or more.

Nursing Implications.—Sa_{O_2} monitoring was shown to be an important component of patient assessment in the PACU. These findings established pulse oximetry as a standard of care in the authors' institution. Supplemental oxygen is now given for patients who exhibit Sa_{O_2} values less than 92%. However, more research in this area, including a larger sample and more rigorous design, is needed.

Comments: This study arose from common questions in clinical practice: What are the best parameters to use for patient assessment and how should new technology and diagnostics be integrated into that assessment? The authors also questioned a standard that didn't seem to quite "fit" with what they were seeing in clinical practice. These questions were answered by their research study. They indeed found that by using only their previous scoring system, some patients would be discharged from the PACU with low SaO_2 values. A somewhat obvious relationship was also validated—that preoperative SaO_2 values were positively correlated with postoperative values. This gave the PACU team information to assess and intervene proactively with potentially high-risk patients in relation to their oxygenation status in the PACU.

This study highlighted the need to use more than 1 assessment measure for patients. More importantly, this study led to the development of a revised standard of care for patients. Although I would argue that more data is needed before practice patterns are changed, this is certainly a first step in that direction. Now, what is needed next? To name a few examples: a larger sample size, different patient populations (especially children), outcome measures of patients who receive supplemental oxygen, and measurement of type of anesthesia used, postoperative medications, and preoperative illnesses.

Of note is the important point the authors made of clinical versus statistical significance. They would have missed an important issue if they had not been able to look beyond the statistics and see valuable clinical trend information.—S. Wingate, RN, DNSc, CCRN, CS

Prolonged Paralysis After Treatment With Neuromuscular Junction Blocking Agents

Gooch JL, Suchyta MR, Balbierz JM, Petajan JH, Clemmer TP (Univ of Utah; LDS Hosp, Salt Lake City)

Crit Care Med 19:1125–1131, 1991 2–5

Problem.—Prolonged paralysis may occur in critically ill patients treated with neuromuscular junction blocking agents. A group of such patients were analyzed.

Methods.—Twelve intensive care unit patients who experienced severe weakness after discontinuation of neuromuscular junction blocking agents were examined. They had a variety of diagnoses, most commonly adult respiratory distress syndrome. Six patients underwent electrodiagnostic studies, and 2 patients underwent muscle biopsy to evaluate neuromuscular transmission.

Findings.—In each patient, muscle weakness was pronounced, but there was no sensory loss. Failure of neuromuscular transmission was noted on both electrodiagnostic studies and muscle biopsy. Most of the patients received medications such as methylprednisolone or gentamicin or had disorders that affect the neuromuscular system; however, none of these was common to all patients. It took several months for patients to recover, and most of them were slow to wean from mechanical ventilation.

Conclusions.—Neuromuscular blocking agents have the potential to cause neurogenic atrophy by blocking neuromuscular transmission. Affected patients require long hospitalization, and their weaning problems appear to be caused by the weakness itself. These drugs must be used cautiously, and patients with poor kidney or liver function must be monitored closely. There does appear to be a dose relationship, therefore, it would be prudent to minimize doses.

Comments: The use of neuromuscular blocking agents such as pancuronium bromide (Pavulon) and vercuronium bromide (Norcuron) is common in critical care units. By blocking the nerve impulse to the muscle, a chemical paralysis is created that paralyzes the intercostal and diaphragm muscles to allow a mechanical ventilator to control the respiratory rate and depth. This therapy prevents the patient from "fighting against" the ventilator and is beneficial in decreasing the work of breathing and improving gas exchange. The standard of practice is to give diazepam (Valium) or morphine sulfate with the neuromuscular blocking agent to decrease sensation so that the patient will not perceive the paralysis.

Given the benefits of drug therapy, we must be aware of the risks also. We know that use of neuromuscular blocking agents prevents assessment of neurologic status. Antagonists such as pyridostigmine bromide (Regonol), neostigmine, or edrophonium, however, can reverse the effects of the blocking agent or the patient can be allowed to "come out from under the effects" of the blocking agent so that the neurologic status can be assessed.

This article warns of another risk of neuromuscular blocking agents in 12 patients, that of prolonged paralysis or weakness. The patients in this study received the blocking agents from 2 to 45 days, with an average of 14.5 days. Whereas the outcome of these patients will not prevent the use of blocking agents, it can explain some of the difficulties patients encounter during their recovery. For example, prolonged weaning from mechanical ventilation may be attributed to the use of blocking agents. Ambulation also may be prolonged due to muscle weakness from the effects of these agents. It seem these drugs are valuable for maintaining respiratory status during acute illness, then may become a nemesis during the recovery phase.—S.F. Wilson, PhD, RN

Persistence of Supply Dependency of Oxygen Uptake at High Levels of Delivery in Adult Respiratory Distress Syndrome.

Clarke C, Edwards JD, Nightingale P, Mortimer AJ, Morris J (University Hospital of South Manchester, England)

Crit Care Med 19:497–502, 1991 2–6

Problem.—Reports of anesthetized patients before and after aortocoronary bypass grafting have shown that oxygen consumption by the tissues seems to be independent of the delivery of oxygen at a critical level. However, these results cannot be applied to critically ill patients with adult respiratory distress syndrome (ARDS). A trial was conducted to determine whether there are any plateaus in oxygen consumption when oxygen delivery is increased in patients with ARDS.

Methods.—Twenty patients aged 18–78 years were investigated. In all patients, ARDS was observed during their stay in the intensive care unit. Many measurements were obtained for each patient. Mathematical models were fitted to data from individuals and to pooled data from all patients.

Findings.—Oxygen delivery ranged from 212 to 1550 mL/min$\cdot$m^2. The variations among patients were great, therefore, it was not justifiable to describe a relationship for the pooled data. The best regression model was linear in 13 patients, cubic in 4 patients, and either cubic or linear in 1 patient (Figs 2–2 and 2–3). No significant relationship could be identified in 2 patients. The relationship between delivery and oxygen consumption for the group was best described by linear regression.

Conclusions.—These patients had no evidence of a plateau in oxygen consumption, even though high levels of oxygen delivery were achieved in all patients. Further research is needed to try to identify a plateau of oxygen consumption at even higher levels of delivery.

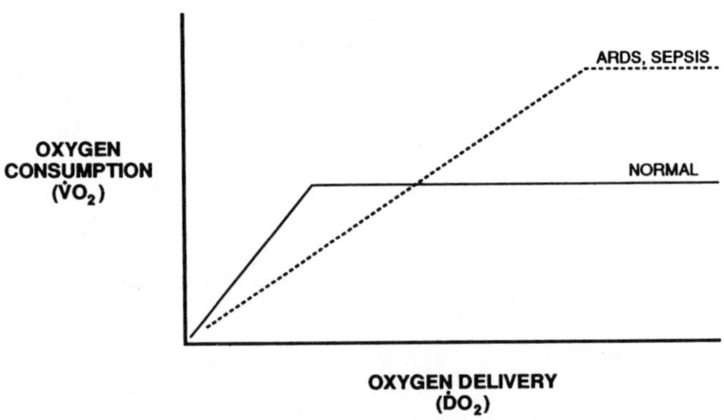

Fig 2–2.—Classic oxygen delivery/oxygen consumption relationship as described in animal models and in ARDS and sepsis. (Courtesy of Clarke C, Edwards JD, Nightingale P, et al: *Crit Care Med* 19:497–502, 1991.)

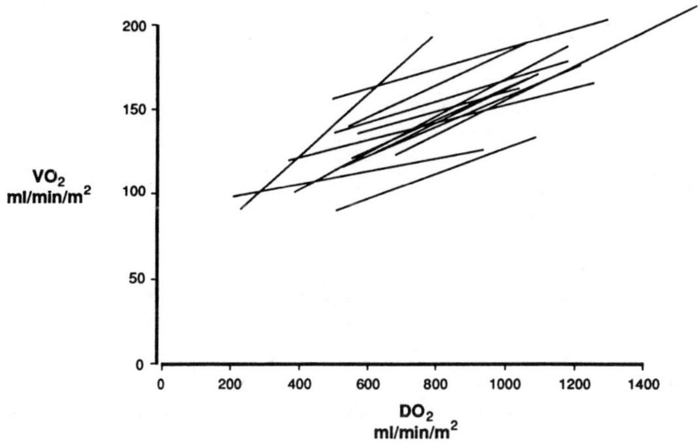

Fig 2–3.—Lines of best fit as determined by simple linear regression in 13 patients. (Courtesy of Clarke C, Edwards JD, Nightingale P, et al: *Crit Care Med* 19:497–502, 1991.)

Comments: This is one in a series of articles in the past decade addressing the concept of oxygen consumption (Vo_2) being dependent on oxygen delivery (Do_2) at a critical point in cellular oxygenation. Although this article has limitations similar to those of articles that preceded it (e.g., limited sample size), the authors point out a potentially important observation. These authors note the lack of a clear point establishing Vo_2 independence from Do_2.

In theory, Vo_2 and Do_2 are independent of each other, resulting in a plateau level (Fig 2–2). When cellular hypoxia is developing, Vo_2 becomes dependent upon Do_2 (the 45 degree slope line in Figure 2–2), reflecting cells might have a higher oxygen need than can be supplied by the blood. Vo_2 becomes dependent upon Do_2 because cells do not receive or use oxygen appropriately. Reasons for the failure of cells to use oxygen range from obstruction of capillary blood flow secondary to microembolization to an inability of mitochondria to chemically process oxygen. When cells cannot receive or use oxygen, the oxygen demand of the cells will exceed oxygen used (consumed). When demand exceeds consumption, Vo_2 becomes dependent upon Do_2. Whatever the cause of Vo_2 to become dependent on Do_2, claims have been made that increasing Do_2 and Vo_2 until they become independent of each other should be a goal in managing hypoxic patients. If Do_2 is increased, hopefully cells that are hypoxic will have blood supply reestablished, and cells will once again start to consume oxygen. When cellular hypoxia is eliminated, further increases in Do_2 will no longer produce increases in Vo_2. Whereas, theoretically, it is logical to try to push Do_2 until Vo_2 no longer increases, no clear evidence exists in the clinical setting that establishes the relationship (as seen in Figure 2–2). This study points out that no plateau level was found that would indicate that Vo_2 became independent of Do_2 as treatment to increase Do_2 was given. From this study, increasing Do_2 did not result in achieving the goal of identifying a point where cellular hypoxia was potentially relieved.

The important point of this article is that it serves to illustrate a need for continued research in the area of assessing clinical hypoxia. Until this research is performed, the practicing nurse must use all available aspects assessing oxygenation, including both Do_2 (e.g., cardiac output, hemoglobin and Sao_2) and Vo_2 measurements. In addition, the use of parameters such as Svo_2, Pvo_2, and lactate levels must be incorporated to aid in determining which patients are at risk for clinical hypoxia.—T. Ahrens, RN, DNS, CCRN

Pressure Controlled Inverse Ratio Ventilation in Respiratory Failure

Briones TL (Univ of Michigan, Ann Arbor)

Dimens Crit Care Nurs 10:254–261, 1991 2–7

Problem.—Determining the proper management of patients with respiratory failure continues to be challenging and controversial. The medical community has searched for optimal mechanical ventilation attuned to different degrees of pulmonary involvement. Pressure controlled inverse ratio ventilation is a ventilatory modality in which the conventional inspiratory-to-expiratory ratio is reversed. Inverse ratio ventilation permits stabilization of pulmonary units and diffusion of gases.

Nursing Assessment and Intervention.—Critical care nurses must have an in-depth understanding of IRV, the indications for its use, and potential complications so that they can make rapid, accurate assessments and intervene when necessary. The first nursing responsibility for patients on IRV is patient comfort. The hyperinflated lung produces a feeling of fullness and can be uncomfortable, resulting in patient anxiety and restlessness. This increases the patient's work of breathing and oxygen consumption. Sedatives or neuromuscular blocking agents are usually needed to ensure patient comfort and compliance. Morphine sulfate and midazolam (Versed) have yielded good results. A continuous intravenous drip is better than an intermittent intravenous push in maintaining steady blood levels and assuring patient comfort. Critical care nurses also assess airway patency in patients undergoing IRV. Standard endotracheal tubes or tracheostomy tubes, preferably with a large diameter, can be used. Tube cuffs should be inflated to minimum leak. Nurses must evaluate airway clearance. Suctioning to clear the airways is limited to short passes and is based on assessment results. A closed suction system usually is recommended. Nurses must take care to ensure that expiration is not impeded by the catheter during suctioning. Critical care nurses assess ventilator settings, making sure that alarms are functional and turned on at all times and closely monitoring and recording airway pressure, rate, tidal volume, and fraction of inspired oxygen. Critical care nurses also continuously monitor the hemodynamic status and arterial blood gases.

Conclusions.—When caring for patients on IRV, the nurse provides comfort, assessment, and preventive measures to help the patient tolerate ventilation and to prevent complications. Collaboration with the respiratory therapist and physician is also essential.

Recommendations.—The following research questions are in need of further investigation:

- Will early initiation of IRV improve mortality rate in patients with respiratory failure?
- What is the incidence of auto-positive end-expiratory pressure in patients on IRV?
- What is the incidence of tachycardia in patients on IRV?
- Is IRV beneficial in patients who have a tendency to retain carbon dioxide (CO_2)?

Comments: The management of severe oxygenation disturbances of a pulmonary origin has not changed appreciably in the past decade. One new method that has developed over the past few years is pressure controlled inverse ratio ventilation (PC-IRV). In this article, a brief review of the concept as well as related research articles on the topic is provided. The author provides simple indications for PC-IRV and nursing implications. The primary value of PC-IRV is the improvement in gas exchange. This improvement is the result of a reduction in intrapulmonary shunting and the subsequent improvement in Pao_2 and Sao_2 values. One area of importance that is not addressed in the article is that, although PC-IRV can improve pulmonary oxygenation, the overall effect on tissue oxygenation has not been shown. Patients with low Pao_2/Sao_2 values do not necessarily die or have increased morbidity. Although it is important to develop therapies that improve pulmonary oxygenation, it is important to remember many of the conditions that cause severe pulmonary dysfunction are multifactorial. Treatment of one aspect (i.e., pulmonary function) without treating the other organ systems may not have any major impact on overall patient outcome. Studies evaluating newer technologies such as PC-IRV also must investigate the impact on patient outcome.—T. Ahrens, RN, DNS, CCRN

Weaning From Mechanical Ventilation: Current Controversies

Knebel AR (Univ of California, San Francisco)

Heart Lung 20:321–334, 1991 2–8

Problem.—Weaning patients with preexisting lung disease from mechanical ventilation can be very difficult. This process is often very lengthy. The process of weaning from mechanical ventilation was reviewed.

Preweaning Phase.—The decision of whether to wean the patient is made in the preweaning phase. The determination of whether a patient is physiologically ready to be weaned is based on reversal of precipitants, CNS assessment, metabolic assessment, cardiovascular and hemodynamic assessment, renal assessment, and pulmonary assessment (table).

Bedside Pulmonary Function Parameters for Predicting Weaning

		Mechanics	
Oxygenation	*Ventilation*	*Strength*	*Endurance*
FIO_2 <0.5 to maintain PaO_2 >50 mm Hg	$\dot{V}E$ requirement <10 L/min	MIP <−25 cm H_2O	MVV >2 × $\dot{V}E$
	VDS/VT <0.55	VC >10 ml/kg	Static compliance >30 ml/cm H_2O
	$PaCO_2$ <60 mm Hg	VT >5 ml/kg	

Abbreviations: MIP, maximal inspiratory pressure; MVV, maximal voluntary ventilation; VC, vital capacity; VDS/VT, dead space to tidal volume ratio; VE, minute volume; VT, tidal volume, $PaCO_2$, partial pressure of carbon dioxide; FIO_2.
Note: Data is compiled from Marini JJ, Wheeler A. *Critical Care—the Essentials*. Baltimore: Williams and Wilkins, 1989:85–96 and Pierson D: *Respir Care* 28:646–662, 1983.
(Courtesy of Knebel AR: *Heart Lung* 20:321–334, 1991.)

The patient also must be psychologically ready to be weaned. Because psychologic stress can precipitate shortness of breath and possibly weaning failure, fear and anxiety must be prevented or reduced. Nurses must establish means of communication with patients so that patients can relay their feelings during weaning.

Weaning Phase.—The most commonly used weaning methods are the T-piece and intermittent mandatory ventilation techniques. The method of weaning is not a significant issue for patients undergoing short-term ventilation. Evidence is inconclusive about which is better for patients with long-term ventilation. Pressure support ventilation is a relatively new method of weaning in which a set level of airway pressure is delivered, augmenting the tidal volume, with the patient controlling the length, depth, and timing of the inspiratory cycle. Another weaning method is continuous positive airway pressure, applying continuous positive pressure to the airway during spontaneous breathing trials with the ventilator.

Extubation Phase.—After successful weaning, the artificial airway must be removed. The primary indicator of successful extubation is the patient's ability to tolerate spontaneous ventilation.

Comments: Weaning from mechanical ventilation is a tremendously important concept in the care of the critically ill. Unfortunately, no one method has been shown to be superior to others in weaning a patient from mechanical ventilation. In this paper, the author addresses many of the major issues in weaning from mechanical ventilation. One of the first issues discussed is that almost any weaning method is effective in the patient who is ready to wean. Determining which method is best becomes a problem, however, in the group of patients who have failed a weaning trial. Once a patient has failed a simple weaning trial, then the selection of a specific weaning plan is necessary. As presented in this paper, T-piece trials and intermittent mandatory ventilation are the most commonly used techniques. To improve the weaning process, pressure support ventilation can be used to reduce the work of breathing or continuous positive airway pressure can be used to maintain oxygenation. *When* these techniques are to be applied, however, is not clear. Because of a lack of clear research supporting a particular weaning technique, hospitals across the country vary widely on their techniques. The author lists in the table common parameters that should be present before beginning a spontaneous trial, yet these parameters are not always accurate. Because of the lack of sensitivity of current weaning parameters, it is not surprising that variations in weaning practices are common across the country. Perhaps the most important thing to remember in the weaning process is the involvement of the critical care nurse. The nurse responsible for managing the care of the patient will be in the best position to evaluate the response to whatever method is used. The nurse also has the responsibility, however, to apply concepts that are beyond simple assessment. In other words, use of simple concepts such as how the patient looks or what the respiratory rate is may not be appropriate. This article provides a framework for the nurse to build a more sophisticated knowledge base to evaluate the method used in weaning.—T. Ahrens, RN, DNS, CCRN

3 Trauma

A Head-Injured Patient: Caloric Needs, Clinical Progress and Nursing Care Priorities

Godbole KB, Berbiglia VA, Goddard L (Southwest Texas Methodist Hosp; Univ of Texas, San Antonio)

J Neurosci Nurs 23:290–294, 1991

3–1

Problem.—In head-injured patients, associated hypermetabolism may affect outcome if the patient's nutritional needs are not assessed and met. The nursing care of the head-injured patient was reviewed to identify appropriate outcomes in terms of nutritional status, skin breakdown, and infection.

Nursing Assessment.—The nurse determines the adequacy of the patient's nutritional status by calculating calorie intake and comparing it to the predicted total energy expenditure, which takes into account both activity and injury. The hypermetabolism seen in many types of injuries is particularly severe in patients with head trauma; their calorie use may resemble that of patients with burns over 30% of their bodies, which may cause malnutrition, infection, impaired skin integrity, and decreased level of consciousness. Initiation of intravenous hyperalimentation within 2 days appears to improve outcome. The first step in preventing malnutrition is interpreting the patient's physiological behavior, such as weight loss, negative nitrogen balance, and decreasing albumin levels.

Nursing Intervention.—Early dietary consultation must be obtained and the patient should be weighed each day. Nursing care may be improved by inservice education on the increased metabolic demands of head-injured patients. Calorimetry may provide a useful basis for nutritional support. Daily interventions include estimating nutrient needs, providing nutritional support, documenting nutrition delivered, noting skin condition, recognizing the risk of infection and skin breakdown, and monitoring blood and urine values. Laboratory values of inadequate nutrition include serum albumin of less than 3.5 g/dL and a total lymphocyte count of less than 1,500 mm^3.

Conclusion.—The increased metabolic demands of head-injured patients affect their nursing care. Primary nursing care priorities may include alteration in cerebral tissue perfusion, potential for injury, and alteration in skin integrity.

Comments: When head-injured patients are admitted to a critical care unit, establishing and maintaining both an effective airway and cerebral perfusion are the priorities. Actually for *any* trauma or burn patient the priorities are airway, breathing, and circulation. Nutrition is low on the priority list. We may not be concerned with nutrition first, but we must be concerned about it within the first 48 hours of admission. Consider the massive amount of inflammation occurring in the body after trauma or burns. There is increased capillary permeability at all sites of injury, leading to edema. This edema is fluid that has left the intravascular spaces and has entered the interstitial spaces, contributing to a fluid deficit. Fluid containing protein is lost from wounds, lowering the serum albumin. Leukocytes, including lymphocytes, are racing to the injured areas to phagocytize foreign substances. All of these activities require energy to run the inflammatory process. Additionally, the fluids and proteins must be replaced. Nutrition is needed in the form of parenteral fluids containing 50% dextrose and amino acids with vitamins and minerals initially to fuel the "fire" in the body created by the body's response to tissue injury. When bowel sounds return, enteral feedings may begin to assist in tissue repair.

Part of the routine assessment must include nutrition. At the very least, note what intravenous fluid is being infused. A liter of 5% dextrose provides about 200 calories. Just comparing that to the 2,000 to 3,000 calories we eat each day will tell us that orders for feeding these patients are needed. The clinical dietitian is a valuable colleague in calculating the number of calories needed and recommending the best way to meet the need. By providing the body with the fuel it needs, it can make more lymphocytes to fight infection and repair more tissue to prevent skin breakdown and enhance healing. Feeding the patient adequately early may prevent prolonged hospitalization resulting from complications of infection and skin breakdown.—S.F. Wilson, RN, PhD

Myocardial Contusion: Using the Index of Suspicion for Assessing Blunt Chest Trauma

Bartlett R (VA Med Ctr, Memphis)

Dimens Crit Care Nurs 10:133–139, 1991 3–2

Problem.—Monitoring patients who incur blunt chest trauma is important for assessing the cause and extent of cardiac trauma. Clinical signs are often difficult to recognize and interpret.

Pathophysiology.—Although histopathologically myocardial contusion bears some resemblance to myocardial infarction, the zone of injury is well demarcated from normal myocardium, and necrosis usually is limited to specific muscle bundles. Sudden deceleration and compression can produce myocardial contusion, or indirect force such as a crush injury of the lower extremities may be responsible.

Nursing Assessment.—Precordial pain may closely mimic that caused by myocardial ischemia or infarction, but it is not relieved by coronary vasodilators (table). Close examination of the torso may show penetration from debris, contusion, deformity, or asymmetric chest wall motion.

Components of Index of Suspicion

Identification of Mechanism of Injury
- **Sudden Deceleration**
  - Motor vehicle accident
  - Use of seatbelts
  - Crushed steering wheel
  - Ejection from vehicle
- **Compression**
  - Animal kick
  - Thrust from flying object
- **Indirect Forces**
  - Crush injury to lower extremities

Performance of Physical Assessment
- **Subjective Data**
  - Precordial chest pain
  - Dyspnea
  - Syncope
- **Objective Data**
  - Assessment of mentation
  - Observation for penetrations, contusions, deformities, paradoxical motion, skin color, and capillary refill
  - Palpation for instability, tenderness, vibration and skin temperature
  - Symmetry of chest movement
  - Rate, rhythm, depth, and effort of breathing
  - Ascultation for murmurs, gallops, or rubs
  - Calculation of urine output

Integration of Diagnostic Reports
- **EKG**
  - Dysrhythmia
  - ST-T wave abnormalities
  - Prolonged QTc
- **CK-MB Elevation**
- **ECHO**
  - Wall motion abnormalities
  - Valvular competency
  - Tamponade
  - Intracardiac thrombi
  - Ejection fraction

Abbreviations: EKG, electrocardiogram; *CK-MB,* creatine phosphokinase-MB; *ECHO,* echocardiography.
(Courtesy of Bartlett R: *Dimers Crit Care Nurs* 10:133–139, 1991.)

The chest is palpated for instability or tenderness. Diagnostic studies include the assay for creatine phosphokinase-MB and 2-dimensional echocardiography. Ongoing assessment is the most important nursing measure in caring for patients who incur blunt chest trauma. Use of an index of suspicion scale, similar to the Glasgow Coma Scale, will help quantify the potential for developing cardiac embarrassment.

Recommendations.—The following clinical research questions are in need of investigation:

- Can an index of suspicion scale be a valid and reliable predictor of symptomatic myocardial contusion?
- What monitoring protocol will be most reliable for assessing perfusion in the patient with blunt chest trauma without disrupting rest?
- How can the index of suspicion be altered to facilitate assessment of the obtunded or unconscious patient?

Comments: A key ingredient in critical care nursing assessment of the trauma patient is an informed index of suspicion to delineate subtle injuries or quickly identify evolving complications. Research on the epidemiology and injury trajectory of the often unpredictable myocardial contusion is sufficient that a nursing protocol including time frames can be established. The author outlines essential monitoring for myocardial contusion. Recent evidence suggests that after 24 hours of intensive care unit monitoring and another 24 hours in telemetry, patients may be discharged home if no other injury is present (1). The assessment plan therefore should be targeted appropriately to the key areas highlighted by the author.—D. Fontaine, RN, DNSc, CCRN

Reference

1. Miller FB, Schumate CR, Richardson JD: Myocardial contusion: When can the diagnosis be eliminated? *Arch Surg* 124:805–808, 1989.

Non-Operative Management of Blunt Splenic Trauma: A 10-Year Experience

Koury HI, Peschiera JL, Welling RE (Good Samaritan Hosp, Cincinnati; Univ of Cincinnati)

Injury 22:349–352, 1991 3–3

Problem and Study Methods.—Patients with traumatic splenic injuries generally have been treated with splenectomy in spite of the relatively high mortality and morbidity rates. Knowledge of the immune function of the spleen and the risk for overwhelming postsplenectomy infection have prompted attempts at splenic salvage. To identify the patient population that can be safely treated nonoperatively, data on 91 patients treated for splenic injuries in 1978–1988 were studied retrospectively; 68 underwent operative therapy and 23 were treated nonoperatively. The operative group had hemodynamic instability and/or peritoneal signs and underwent exploratory laparotomy. The nonoperative group was diagnosed by CT (20) or by liver/spleen scans and peritoneal lavage (3).

Findings.—All patients in the nonoperative group had upper quadrant abdominal pain and tenderness; 3 had associated left rib fractures and 2 had abdominal injuries. Blood transfusions were necessary in 6 patients. All were admitted to the intensive care unit and monitored with serial abdominal examinations and hemoglobin estimations. These patients had an average hospital stay of 8 days and were instructed to restrict strenuous physical activity for 2–3 months after discharge. Splenectomy was performed on 2 patients after unsuccessful nonoperative therapy.

Conclusion.—Splenectomy should be performed in patients with severe multisystem trauma or penetrating abdominal trauma and in those who require more than 4 units of blood over a 48-hour period. Hemodynamically stable patients can be evaluated by CT and closely monitored during their hospital stay. Selected patients can be safely treated nonoperatively with adequate nursing care and rest.

Comments: Despite all the complexities of trauma care, it is fascinating that the spleen can create such controversy. The treatment of hemodynamically stable blunt splenic trauma is controversial. Because some of the controversy revolves around astute critical care observation, it naturally becomes an issue for critical care nurses. What is the nature of the controversy? What are the critical care nursing roles?

This topic is important because of the frequency in which the spleen is injured in blunt abdominal trauma. There has been controversy surrounding the evolution of aggressive vs. conservative approaches in splenic trauma. This is typified by splenectomy to splenorrhaphy to now in the 1990s, nonoperative splenic trauma management in "selected" patients. The controversy pits those who believe in the seriousness of the threat of overwhelming postsplenectomy infection in the asplenic patient against those who are concerned that a conservative approach, nonoperative management, may miss injuries, lead to an increased risk of blood transfusion related hepatitis, or promote the possibility of delayed splenic rupture. Lucas pointed out that the true delayed splenic rupture rate is 1% (1).

This article is one of a growing number suggesting that, in carefully selected patients, observation and careful monitoring can substitute for exploratory surgery. Patient exclusions include any who are hemodynamically unstable or not mentally alert. Because of the key role of surveillance, critical care nurses have a major function.

Growing support for nonoperative management of the adult spleen has not reached the acceptance it has with splenic injury in children (2). However, we have witnessed an historical change in the view of the spleen from an organ with little merit to one that is possibly essential for life (1). The role of the spleen in defense against infections is now well appreciated.

Nursing care after a CT scan of the abdomen and a decision to sit tight and monitor an abdominal trauma patient with a minor splenic injury includes explaining to the patient and family the need for frequent abdominal assessments and eliciting the patient's willingness to confirm any increasing tenderness. When tenderness worsens during monitoring, surgery is indicated. Mental status must remain intact for this strategy to be useful. Hemodynamics must be vigorously assessed and hematocrit checked every 6 hours. Bed rest for 7 days has been advocated with the goal of allowing the spleen to heal itself. The magic of 7 days has not been systematically investigated.

Patient education regarding no strenuous activity for 6–8 weeks and no contact sports for 6 months must be communicated. Nurses must investigate the philosophy of splenic trauma care for their institution. Further research will help delineate inclusion criteria for conservative therapy, and future guidelines can dictate what activities can be performed safely by the patient to speed the discharge process.—D. Fontaine, RN, DNSc, CCRN

References

1. Lucas C: Splenic trauma: Choice of management. *Ann Surg* 213:98–112, 1991.
2. Wilson RH, Moorehead RJ: Management of splenic trauma. *Injury* 23:5–9, 1992.

The Spectrum of Abdominal Injuries Associated With the Use of Seat Belts

Rutledge R, Thomason M, Oller D, Meredith W, Moylan J, Clancy T, Cunningham P, Baker C (Univ of North Carolina, Charlotte; Bowman Gray School of Medicine; Duke Univ; New Hanover Mem Hosp; East Carolina School of Medicine; et al)

J Trauma 31:820–826, 1991 3–4

Problem.—Trauma remains the most common cause of death in children and adults younger than 40. Seat belts are demonstrably effective in reducing morbidity and deaths from motor vehicle crashes, but injuries from seat belt use have been described. The range of abdominal injuries incurred in motor vehicle accidents in belted and unbelted occupants was examined. Data were available for 3,901 victims.

Data Points for Belted and Unbelted Patients

VARIABLE	BELTED	UNBELTED
Number of Patients	1,733	2,168
Age	37.4+19.1	29.3+16
Gender (male/female)	947/786 (54.6%/45.4%)	1,389/779 (64.1%/35.9%)*
Position in Car (driver/passenger)	696/447 (60.9%/39.1%)	729/700 (51.0%/49.0%)*
Abdominal Injuries (Y/N)	240 (13.9%)	291 (13.4%)
Splenic Injuries	77 (4.4%)	118 (5.4%)
Other Abdominal Injuries	63 (2.6%)	95 (4.3%)
Hepatic Injuries	65 (3.8%)	87 (4.0%)
Gastrointestinal Injuries	59 (3.4%)	38 (1.8%)*
Renal Injuries	41 (2.4%)	49 (2.3%)
Bladder	19 (1.1%)	26 (1.2%)
Diaphragm	15 (0.9%)	16 (0.9%)
Pancreas	2 (0.1%)	6 (0.3%)
Lumbar Spine Injuries	91 (5.3%)	108 (5.0%)
Blood Pressure	128+29	125+29
Pulse	93.5+22.5	97+26
Respirations	22+7.6	21+8.5
Scene Trauma Score	14.6+2.4	13.4+3.3
ED Trauma Score	15.1+2.2	14.2+3.1
Admission Hct.	38.7+6.8	38.5+7.2
Glasgow Coma Scale	14.0+2.7	12.9+3.4*
Blood Transfused	1.2+3.2	1.7+4.4
AIS Head and Neck	0.9+1.4	1.4+1.7*
AIS Chest	0.9+1.4	0.9+1.4
AIS Abdomen	0.5+1.0	0.46+1.0
AIS Extremities	1.1+1.2	1.1+1.3
Computer Derived ISS	10.8+8.4	13.5+10.2*
Days on Ventilator	2.3+8.3	3.5+9.4*
Days in ICU	4.0+9.5	5.5+10.9*
Days in Hospital	10.2+14.1	13.1+19.7*
Hospital Charges	$11,900+36,600	$16,700+48,900*
Death	59 (3.4%)	121 (5.6%)*

*$P < .01$.
(Courtesy of Rutledge R, Thomason M, Oller D, et al: *J Trauma* 31:820–826, 1991.)

Findings.—Mortality was more than twice as high for unbelted patients as for belted patients (7% vs. 3.2%). Unbelted occupants had more frequent and more severe head injuries. Although the incidence of abdominal injury was similar in these groups, gastrointestinal tract injuries were significantly more prevalent in belted patients (table). Liver and spleen injuries were similarly frequent in the belted and unbelted groups.

Implications.—The "seat belt syndrome" involves injuries in the plane of the lap part of the belt. The colon and small bowel are the primary sites of injury, but the stomach, liver, spleen, and pancreas are occasionally injured. It remains uncertain how often severe seat belt-related injuries occur. Chest injury is more likely when there is an abdominal injury. Even if belt use increases the risk of abdominal injury, it does save lives.

Comments: A key point in discussing seat belt injuries is to reflect that a restraint that keeps an individual in a vehicle is always better than no restraint. The paradox is that while seat belts save lives by keeping individuals in the vehicle and away from the windshield, they may produce abdominal injury. The seat belt syndrome dealing with lap belts was first described in the *Journal of Trauma* in 1962 (1). Today, there is evidence that improperly applied 3-point restraint seat belts may result in injury (2).

Nursing implications based on abdominal trauma resulting from seat belts are twofold: an accurate assessment of events of the injury with a high index of suspicion for occult injury is needed and continued education of patients, family members, and the community is a responsibility. Nurses in the acute resuscitative trauma phase of patient care play a role in thorough injury assessment. This indicates use of all data points, including not only information regarding whether or not seat belts were used, but type of restraint and any indication that it was improperly applied. Open communication with prehospital providers and a willingness to elicit this information from them would be useful in diagnosing potential subtle injuries.

Education of the patient, family, and others is an important concept when we consider that trauma may be a "chronic" disease. Persons admitted with trauma who survive often enter our health care system with trauma again (unbelievable, but true). The first trauma admission, even though a crisis, is a great opportunity to emphasize proper seat belt use and child restraints, if appropriate.

Until air bags or fail proof passive restraint devices are developed and widely adopted, seat belt injuries will occur. We need to keep in perspective that the abdominal trauma patient with a seat belt injury often has a surgically correctable condition, whereas those who are injured and are not wearing seat belts continue to suffer severe head injury and death.—D. Fontaine, RN, DNSc, CCRN

References

1. Garrett JW, Braunstein PW: The seat belt syndrome. *J Trauma* 2:220, 1962.
2. Turnes CI: Improperly positioned passenger-restraint systems as associated mechanisms of injury in motor vehicular collisions. *JEN* 17:373–379, 1991.

Is Early Prediction of Outcome in Severe Head Injury Possible?

Waxman K, Sundine MJ, Young RF (Univ of California, Irvine)
Arch Surg 126:1237–1242, 1991 3–5

Purpose and Study Methods.—Efforts at cost containment and decreasing human suffering would be aided if there were a means of identifying at an early stage those patients with head injury who will die or have devastating disability. A series of 306 head-injured patients whose Glasgow Coma Scale (GCS) scores were 10 or below were reviewed. Initial scores were assigned before patients received sedating or paralyzing agents.

Findings.—Mortality in this series was 38%, and another 8% of patients were discharged in a persistent vegetative state. The initial GCS score did not correlate well with the outcome (table). Scores estimated 6 hours after presentation correlated more closely with the eventual outcome, but many patients with GCS scores as low as 3 had good neurologic recovery. It was not possible to predict outcomes sensitively even when age, associated injuries, blood pressure, the presence of spontaneous ventilation, and CT findings were taken into account, despite the fact that of all these factors influenced survival. Patients with initially normal CT findings had the best outlook, but 4% of them died and 23% were discharged with disability.

Implications.—Aggressive treatment should not be denied to patients solely on the basis of the initial GCS score. Any cost savings are offset by the risk of a patient who could have a good outcome dying or incurring

Initial Scores on the Glasgow Coma Scale Related to Outcome

		Outcome Score, % of Patients*				
Initial Score	No. of Patients	1	2	3	4	5
3	117	75	7	5	3	10
4	36	39	19	25	8	8
5	19	17	22	30	None	31
6	36	11	8	33	22	25
7	40	10	2	13	30	45
8	20	10	None	25	15	50
9	14	None	None	7	21	72
10	24	4	None	8	20	68

* An outcome score of *1* indicates death; 2, vegetative state; 3, severe disability; 4, moderate disability; and 5, good recovery. Percentages may not total 100 because of rounding.

(Courtesy of Waxman K, Sundine MJ, Young RF: *Arch Surg* 126:1237–1242, 1991.)

unnecessary disability. Most deaths occur within 2 days. Aggressive treatment is recommended until outcome is clear, at which point treatment options should be discussed with family members.

Comments: This study should stimulate great collaborative, ethical discussion among trauma team members in critical care settings. The bad news is no, we cannot predict outcome in patients with severe head injury before 6 hours after injury. The good news is that some patients make a dramatic recovery despite low GCS scores and multiple abnormalities seen on CT scan. Or is this "good news"? All critical care nurses have anecdotes of the devastating nature of head injuries despite the occasional *National Enquirer* description of a coma patient who awakens after months to a lick from a family dog. These authors recognize that their belief in aggressive treatment for all head-injured patients is a controversial one and raises several questions.

Questions to consider include how "good" is a good recovery after severe head injury? What about the existence of cognitive rehabilitation programs? Typically, few patients receive this effective service. Is unrealistic optimism of families or health care providers a problem? Mirr's study of family members' concerns in severe head injury suggests that inability to predict outcomes and the accompanying uncertainty is very stressful for family members who are expected to be decision-makers (1). Despite discussing discontinuing life support, these family members were concerned over the feeling of abandoning the patient or giving up hope. And, finally, at what point will society and the health care community together look at costs and limited resources?

No other traumatic injury creates more disabling long-term effects on quality of life than head injury. The search for early outcome predictors of severe head injury must continue for reasons of scarce resource allocation, cost containment, and most importantly, patient and family suffering. Choi and colleagues have developed a prediction tree based on 23 factors that may hold promise for future research in head injury (2). The Traumatic Coma Data Bank offers an excellent resource for the study of outcome in severe head injury and for the development of prognostic models (3).

Nurses who care for severely head-injured patients must listen to family members and, as realistically as possible, answer questions. Until we have predictive models for head-injured patients to guide our critical care counseling, nurses will need to support families in their decisions and work to make cognitive rehabilitation more of a national priority for these patients. Encouraging helmet wearing on motorcycles and bicycles also will make critical care nurses feel more useful in preventing the tragedy of severe head injury.—D. Fontaine, RN, DNSc, CCRN

References

1. Mirr MP: Factors affecting decisions made by family members of patients with severe head injury. *Heart Lung* 20:228–235, 1991.
2. Choi SC, Muizelaar JP, Barnes TY, et al.: Prediction tree for severely head-injured patients. *J Neurosurg* 75:251–255, 1991.

3. Foulkes MA, Eisenberg HM, Jane JA, et al: The Traumatic Coma Data Bank: Design, methods, and baseline characteristics. *J Neurosurg* 75:S8–S13, 1991.

Traumatic Injury During Pregnancy

Oakley LE, Johnson JD (Maury Regional Hosp, Columbia, Tenn)

Crit Care Nurse 11:64–72, 1991 3–6

Problem.—Various changes that accompany pregnancy, such as altered balance and gait and the enlarging abdomen itself, predispose pregnant women to traumatic injury. An estimated 6% to 7% of pregnant women will be injured. Nurses have a responsibility to optimize the outcome for both the woman and her fetus.

Types of Injury.—Fetal injury is most frequent later in pregnancy when the amniotic fluid volume is lower relative to the mass of the fetus. Motor vehicle accidents are the chief cause of blunt trauma in pregnancy, followed by falls. Falls are the most common cause of minor injury. Penetrating injuries appear to have a predilection for the pregnant abdomen in late gestation. Extensive burn injuries are rare. Pregnancy is a cause of domestic violence and can trigger physical abuse.

Nursing Interventions.—The plan of care for the pregnant trauma patient is outlined in the table. Any female trauma victim of child-bearing age should be considered pregnant until proved otherwise. The obviously pregnant trauma victim is placed in the left lateral decubitus position to limit pressure on the vena cava. Supplemental high-flow oxygen is given to all injured pregnant women. A complete radiologic workup is appropriate to avoid the risk of injury going undetected. A urinalysis is done, and a complete blood count and clotting studies are obtained.

Comments: The dramatic emotional overlay of the injured pregnant patient makes the nursing care of these 2 patients an exciting challenge. This review illustrates how timely care for the mother helps to assure fetal survival whenever possible. Because trauma nurses do not encounter this situation frequently, the nursing diagnosis and collaborative problem format used in this review will be very useful to focus needed interventions.

Psychosocial and family care is emphasized equally with the collaborative physiologic problems. Nurses are never more skilled than in dealing with critical illness and emotionally overwhelming concerns like untimely mother or fetal death. When outcomes are poor for the fetus, who works more closely with the mother as the grieving process begins? Clearly, the critical care nurse is the one consistent presence. This is a plan of care that should be kept in any emergency setting or critical care unit where pregnant trauma patients may be admitted.—D. Fontaine, RN, DNSc, CCRN

Nursing Plan of Care: Traumatic Injury During Pregnancy

Nursing Diagnoses		Collaborative Problems	
Alteration in comfort: Pain related to:	**Injury and/or surgical procedures** - position for comfort Comfort measures such as back rubs and application of heat or cold as appropriate Decrease environmental stimuli such as noise and light Judicious use of pain medications with attention to pregnancy category	**Alterations in CO related to:**	**Vena cava syndrome:** reposition patient on left side or on back with 15 pelvic tilt to the left **Decreased blood volume:** see fluid volume deficit
Fear/anxiety related to:	**Unexpected hospitalization; uncertain fetal and maternal outcomes** - provide realistic explanations of maternal/fetal injuries and procedures according to level of understanding Encourage verbalization/communication of feelings	**Fluid volume deficit related to:**	**Blood loss:** IV fluid and blood replacement Continuous monitoring of vital signs, CVP, CO Hourly intake and output (including Foley catheter and NG output) Monitor electrolytes and hematocrit as needed Continuous fetal monitoring with obstetric consultation **Burns/electrical injury:** same interventions

(continued)

Table *(continued)*

Nursing Diagnoses		Collaborative Problems	
Alteration in family processes related to:	**Disruption of usual family functioning** - encourage family members to ask questions and verbalize feelings/concerns	**Potential for fetal injury:**	Continuous fetal monitoring for at least 24 to 48 hours after injury
	Facilitate communication between family members		After 48 hours, consider biweekly nonstress tests or biophysical profile
	Involve family members in patient's care as appropriate		Monitor for decreased fetal movement
	Notify clergy as indicated		
Grieving/anticipatory grieving related to:	**Actual or potential death of fetus** Provide realistic explanations of expected outcomes	**Potential for fetal injury:**	Monitor for abruptio placentae, preterm labor, uterine rupture, and rupture of membranes (see Table)
	Encourage expression of feelings		Serial ultrasounds as indicated
			Amniocentesis
	Allow family members to see/ hold stillborn or nonviable infant after birth		Kleihauer-Betke test
	Provide grief packet to parents - footprints, photos, lock of hair, birth certificate		Rh immune globulin for Rh-negative woman with documented fetomaternal hemorrhage or after infusions of Rh-positive blood
	Assist with funeral or other postmortem arrangements		Prevent maternal hypotension

Nursing Diagnoses		Collaborative Problems	
Grieving/anticipatory	**Potential death of mother** Provide realistic explanations of expected outcomes Encourage expression of feelings Allow family members to spend time with the mother before and immediately after her death Assist with funeral or other postmortem arrangements	**Potential for fetal injury:**	Monitor for signs and symptoms of maternal infection Avoid tetracycline, vasoactive drugs, and other medications contraindicated during pregnancy, as previously discussed
Alteration in parenting related to:	**Hospitalization of infant and/or mother** Keep patient and family informed of fetal status Promote attachment, when possible, after delivery Allow contact with other children, when appropriate Provide childbirth classes and appropriate reading material in the convalescent phase		
		Potential for infection:	Monitor temperature every 2 to 4 hours, as indicated Daily WBC count with differential, as indicated

(continued)

Table *(continued)*

Nursing Diagnoses	Collaborative Problems	
	Potential for infection:	Blood, urine, sputum, and wound cultures for unexplained temperature elevations and/or elevated WBC
		Rotate IV sites and replace invasive lines as per hospital protocol
		Tetanus prophylaxis as indicated
		Consider hepatitis and HIV testing
	Alteration in comfort; pain related to:	**Preterm labor** Monitor for contractions
		Position patient on left side
		Consider need for IV fluid bolus
		Use tocolytics such as magnesium sulfate and ritodrine (Yutopar) as indicated
		Prepare for delivery; notify perinatologist and neonatologist
	Alteration in nutrition related to:	**NPO status and increased nutritional demands of pregnancy** - IV hydration, initially

Nursing Diagnoses	Collaborative Problems	
	Alteration in nutrition related to:	**NPO status and increased nutritional demands of pregnancy**
		Monitor for return of bowel sounds, flatus, stool
		Nutrition consult
		Total parenteral nutrition (TPN) or tube feedings, as appropriate
		Daily weights
		Serial laboratory studies as per hospital protocol, including albumin, transferrin, 24 hour urine for urea nitrogen
	Impaired physical mobility related to:	**Severity of injury** - position for comfort, avoiding the supine position
		Consider use of therapeutic bed such as a low airloss bed
		Decrease likelihood of thrombus/embolus formation through use of range of motion exercises and antiembolic stockings

Abbreviations: CO, cardiac output; *CVP*, central venous pressure; *NPO*, nothing by mouth; *WBC*, white blood cell.
(Courtesy of Oakley LE, Johnson JD: *Crit Care Nurs* 11:64–72, 1991.)

Obesity and Increased Mortality in Blunt Trauma

Choban PS, Weireter LJ Jr, Maynes C (Naval Hosp Jacksonville, Fla; Sentara Norfolk Gen Hosp, Norfolk, Va; Virginia Med School, Norfolk)
J Trauma 31:1253–1257, 1991 3–7

Average of Variables for Study Population

Variable	Group: Normal (BMI<27) (n = 140)	Group: Overweight (BMI 27 - 31) (n = 25)	Group: Severely Overweight (BMI>31) (n = 19)	P Value
Age (years)	31.7 ± 1.13	32.7 ± 2.6	39.8 ± 3.25	NS
ISS	21.6 ± 1.3	22.9 ± 2.7	22.7 ± 4.14	NS
LOS (days)	16.7 ± 1.9	14.3 ± 4.31	7.8 ± 1.25	NS
VD (days)	4.3 ± 0.9	3.9 ± 2.4	3.9 ± 1.14	NS
Complications (average patient)	0.50	0.48	0.95*	<0.0001
Mortality (%)	5.0	8.0	42.1*	<0.0001

*Difference significant.
(Courtesy of Choban PS, Weireter LJ, Maynes C: *J Trauma* 31:1253–1257, 1991.)

Problem.—Overweight patients have higher rates of postoperative complications and mortality than do patients of normal weight. The problems of overweight trauma patients were evaluated, and factors that would improve the care of such patients were identified.

Study Methods.—A chart review was made of all blunt trauma patients older than age 12 years admitted to Sentara Norfolk General Hospital between January 1 and July 31, 1987. Of 351 records examined, 184 were found to contain both admission height and weight. The 184 records also were examined for age, gender, mechanism of injury, severity of injury, complications, and outcome. Weight and height were used to calculate body mass index (BMI).

Findings.—The study group included 123 men and 61 women; their average age was 33.66 years, and their average Injury Severity Score (ISS) was 21.87. Based on BMI, 24% were overweight and 10% were severely overweight (more than 31 kg/m^2). The average and overweight groups had similar rates of mortality (5% and 8%, respectively). The severely overweight group, however, had a mortality of 42.1%, an increase not accounted for by a greater ISS. The severely overweight had a higher complication rate, resulting from an increase in pulmonary problems. They also had fewer ventilator days and a shorter hospital stay because of rapid deterioration to death (table). Respiratory distress syndrome hastened death in the severely overweight.

Conclusion.—The overweight state is known to have an adverse effect on health and longevity. Those who are severely overweight have a high mortality after blunt trauma, even with the same interventions given patients of normal weight. The cause of poor outcome in the obese is not fully understood, but it may be related to pulmonary failure and to larger fat depots in adipose tissue.

Comments: Critical care nursing requirements for the obese trauma patient have not been addressed in the literature. With the recognition that obesity and trauma represent the merger of 2 current epidemics, guidelines for the complex management of these patients are needed. Few reports exist to suggest modifications in trauma care that work well with obese patients (1). The authors have demonstrated in a preliminary manner the incidence of obesity and trauma and documented the increased complication rate and mortality in the morbidly obese.

This information will not be surprising to trauma nurses who realize the risky business of delicately balancing critical care therapies in the obese patient. We are all too often operating without scientific basis in caring for these complex patients because many of the principles of trauma care have been developed based on "normal weight" individuals. For example, we believe in the importance of early nutritional therapy in the stressed state of critical illness but may find restrictions of essential nutrients in these patients. Collaboration with the nutritional support team is required, and nutritional status must be evaluated frequently with calculation of caloric need. More research is needed to guide nutritional therapy for the obese critically ill patient.

Positioning is another good example where guidelines need to be established. The tendency to leave the patient who is morbidly obese in one position, although convenient for the health care team, is an unacceptable practice. From a physiological standpoint, the positioning principles that guide critical care nursing practice of the normal-weight patient must be adapted and individualized. According to the authors, these patients have a tendency to develop more pulmonary complications. An appropriate bed needs to be obtained early, and the patient must be positioned for maximum oxygenation/ventilation, skin care, and comfort. This may require choosing the optimal position for a patient in respiratory failure using compliance curves and frequent oxygenation and ventilation assessment based on invasive or noninvasive measures. Is it possible that morbidly obese trauma patients develop more pulmonary complications because we have not developed creative ways to implement these standards?

Primary nursing, patient advocacy, and sensitivity are essential in caring for the obese trauma patient. I will never forget an exemplary primary nurse who was frustrated with the negative, joking remarks of her colleagues, made in the presence of an intubated patient, when she needed their assistance in moving this obese elderly gentleman with multiple fractures. She told everyone outside the patient's room that there would be no further unprofessional comments and wrote this in detail in the care plan. It worked. We need to practice sensitive, caring behaviors with all our patients, especially those who are morbidly obese. We need collaboration with nutritional support and respiratory therapy at a minimum to provide quality care and improve patient outcome for this subgroup of critically ill trauma patients.

The next time a morbidly obese trauma patient enters your unit, why not develop an ongoing critique of the care provided? Ask the following: Are we adequately relieving pain? Is the nutritional support appropriate? Is the patient optimally positioned for oxygenation/ventilation and skin care? Are we all dealing sensitively with the patient and family? Have we obtained the proper size equipment? Based on answers, revise the care delivered to promote excellence in critical care nursing of the morbidly obese trauma patient.—D. Fontaine, RN, DNSc, CCRN

Reference

1. Ochsner M, Herr D, Drucker W, et al: A modified Seldinger technique for peritoneal lavage in trauma patients who are obese. *Surg Gyn Obstet* 173:158–160, 1991.

4 Neurologic Dysfunction

Assessing the Comatose Patient in the Intensive Care Unit
Stewart-Amidei C (La Grange, Ill)
Clin Issues Crit Care Nurs 2:613–622, 1991 4–1

Purpose.—Too little is known about how patients experience coma and about its natural course. Arousal and awareness are inferred phenomena, known only through observed behavioral responses. The anatomy of consciousness and coma assessment is discussed.

Assessment.—In the United States, the Glasgow Coma Scale (GCS) is most commonly used to document coma. The GCS evaluates eye opening, verbal responsiveness, and motor responsiveness. The best responses in these categories are summed up, with a score of 15 indicating full consciousness and a score of 3 indicating deep coma. Any score less than 8 generally means that the patient is comatose. Focal deficits in oculomotor function or in motor or verbal responses are not reflected in the scale. The Reaction Level Scale may be especially useful for bedside

The Reaction Level Scale

Level	*Label*	*Description*
1	Alert	Oriented; if intubated reacts quickly; if sleeping, arouses quickly
2	Drowsy or confused	Responds to light stimuli; reactions are delayed; may be disoriented to time and place
3	Very drowsy or confused	Responds to strong stimuli such as loud noise, shaking, or pain; may respond verbally, or by attempting eye contact, warding off pain, or obeying commands
4	Unconscious, localizes	On painful stimulation of fingertips, other hand moves to push stimuli away
5	Unconscious, withdraws	On painful stimulation of fingertips, pulls stimulated hand away
6	Unconscious, flexion response	Does not localize or withdraw; flexes arms and wrists to stimuli
7	Unconscious, extensor response	Does not localize or withdraw; arms and legs extend to stimuli (if both flexion and extension are noted, best response is recorded)
8	Unconscious, no response to pain	With repeated strong stimulation, no movement noted in face, arms, or legs

(Courtesy of Stewart-Amidei C: *Clin Issues Crit Care Nurs* 2:613–622, 1991.)

monitoring of patients with acute neurologic dysfunction. It consists of 8 categories of consciousness ranging from alertness to unconsciousness with no response to painful stimuli (table). The Reaction Level Scale is at least as sensitive as the GCS and is possibly more sensitive.

Conclusion.—There may be a trend away from describing a level of consciousness and toward describing the level of reaction.

Comments: When I began my nursing practice in the 60s, we assessed coma using adjectives such as alert, lethargic, stuporous, obtunded, semicomatose, and comatose. On the back of the assessment sheet were detailed definitions of these words so that the labeling would be consistent. These descriptors were replaced by the Glasgow Coma Scale, which is quantitative. I have seen this scale used improperly as a neurologic assessment tool instead of as a scale to quantify the degree of coma. The Reaction Level Scale contains some features of both of the above 2 scales. It uses adjectives to label coma as well as a numerical scale (table). The descriptors include data related to the arousal and skeletal motor response. Additional data needed to complete the coma assessment include pupillary reaction, eye movements, and respiratory pattern. I recommend trying this scale to evaluate its effectiveness. Comparisons of the Glasgow Coma Scale and the Reaction Level Scale would provide useful data to apply in clinical practice.

Regardless of the scale used, nurses must document the arousal state of their patients carefully. Remember too that a patient's arousal state changes continually. Just because your assessment is different from the nurse who assessed the patient during the last hour does not necessarily mean that you are in error or that the previous nurse was. If you are unsure of your findings, consult with a colleague. The critical care nurse will be the first person to detect a change in the trend of the patient's state of consciousness and the one to take action when warranted.—S.F. Wilson, RN, PhD

Spinal Cord Injury: Rehabilitation Adds Life to Years

De Vivo MJ, Richards JS, Stover SL, Go BK (Univ of Alabama, Birmingham)

West J Med 154:602–606, 1991 4–2

Purpose.—The National Spinal Cord Injury Statistical Center (NSCISC) database contains information on demographics and medical, vocational, and economic outcomes for persons injured since 1973. This report updates some of the findings published in 1986.

Demographics.—Since 1973, 13,763 patients have been treated at model systems located throughout the nation. The mean age of all patients was 30.5 years; the most common age was 19 years; and 59.3% of patients were 16–30 years of age. Of all patients enrolled inthe NSCISC database, 82.3% were male.

Impairment.—Of the patients, 54.2% had cervical injuries, 35.3% had thoracic injuries, and 10.5% had lumbosacral injuries. Neurologic func-

Change in Degree of Preserved Neurologic Function (Frankel Grade) Between Injury and Discharge From Rehabilitation (n = 4,934)

Frankel Grade	Percent at Injury	Improved	No Change	Declined	Percent at Discharge
Complete (A)	51.9	10.3	89.7	...	47.4
Preserved sensation (B)	13.1	45.2	50.3	4.5	9.3
Motor, nonfunctional (C)	13.1	55.9	41.5	2.6	9.0
Motor, functional (D)	21.9	7.3	90.7	2.0	32.3
Recovery (E)	...	...	...	...	2.0

(Courtesy of De Vivo MJ, Richards JS, Stover SL, et al: *West J Med* 154:602–606, 1991.)

tion was assessed using Frankel's 5-level classification, in which **A** represents no preserved motor or sensory function below the zone of partial preservation, **B** represents preserved sensation only, **C** represents minimal preserved voluntary function that performs no useful purpose, **D** is preserved motor function, and **E** denotes complete recovery of all motor and sensory function.

Recovery.—Assessment of neurologic recovery in 4,934 patients admitted within 24 hours of injury and for whom complete admission and discharge neurologic data were available reveals that 51.9% of patients initially were Frankel grade **A,** 13.1% were Frankel grade **B,** 13.1% were Frankel grade **C,** and 21.9% were Frankel grade **D** (table). Only 10.3% of Frankel grade **A** patients had an improved Frankel grade at discharge, whereas 45.2% of Frankel grade **B** patients and 55.9% of Frankel grade **C** patients had improved at least 1 Frankel grade at discharge. Most Frankel grade **D** patients still had some neurologic impairment at discharge, but most were improved, and 7.3% had complete neurologic recovery. Some patients continued to improve neurologically for 18 months after discharge.

Residence.—Of 13,330 persons who completed rehabilitation, 94.1% went to a private residence in the community, 4% were sent to a nursing home, 1.5% went to another hospital, and .4% went to another destination. Of 1,366 persons who were followed for 10 years, 98% still reside in private residences.

Employment.—Of 6,862 persons aged 16–59 years with known employment status, only 12.6% were employed 2 years after injury, whereas 38.3% were employed by 12 years after injury. Persons re-employed shortly after injury almost always returned to the same job with the same employer, whereas those whose reentry into the job market was delayed usually got a different type of job with a different employer. Significant predictors of re-employment were younger age, male gender, white race, higher educational level, higher motivation, higher functional ability scores, and being employed before injury.

Comments: Invariably when you are caring for a new spinal cord-injured patient, you are asked by a friend or family member, "Is he or she going to be all right?" You have cared for patients like these whose family member will ask, "Will he or she be able to use their arms and legs?" Or perhaps you hear "What will he or she be like following hospital discharge?" The thoughts that run through your head span the gamut from a dependent response such as "the physician can answer those questions for you" to an independent response that proposes hope, but realistic hope. The information in this article can provide some factual data for you. For example, by referring to the first 2 columns in the table, we learn the following: Of the 52% of the 4,934 people reported in a sample who were Frankel grade **A** (no motor or sensory function) on admission, 10.3% had improved at discharge. Of the 13% of the sample who were Frankel grade **B** (no motor, but preserved sensation) at admission, 45% improved at discharge. Even a greater percentage was noted for the patients who were Frankel grade **C** on admission. So, the words of encouragement might be that (1) each patient is unique and progresses at an individual rate, (2) some patients continue to improve for 18 months after discharge, (3) the more extensive the neurologic damage (i.e., those closer to a Frankel grade **A**), the less recovery there may be.

Outcomes can be described in terms of residence and employment. Of the 13,330 persons who completed rehabilitation, 94% were living in a private residence. The employment figures are found in the abstract above. There are federal and state resources to train many spinal cord-injured persons. There is realistic hope for a productive life, but it is a life far different from the one the person experienced before the injury. This adjustment requires a great deal of work for patients and their significant others.

An intriguing thought that this article brings out is that critical care nurses often never learn what happens to these spinal cord-injured persons. Perhaps one aspect of job satisfaction would be to learn the outcome of these people. The critical care unit could request a follow-up report on patients after discharge from the hospital to rehabilitation facilities and then another report after completion of rehabilitation. Many rehabilitation facilities would be happy to provide this follow-up data because it builds positive public relations with the critical care units.—S.F. Wilson, RN, PhD

Autonomic Dysreflexia: A Nursing Challenge in the Care of the Patient With a Spinal Cord Injury

Dunn KL (Dept of VA Med Ctr, San Diego)
J Cardiovasc Nurs 5:57–64, 1991 4–3

Problem.—Autonomic dysreflexia (AD), a recently accepted North American Nursing Diagnosis Association diagnosis, is most frequent and most marked in patients having cord lesions above the T5 level. It occurs

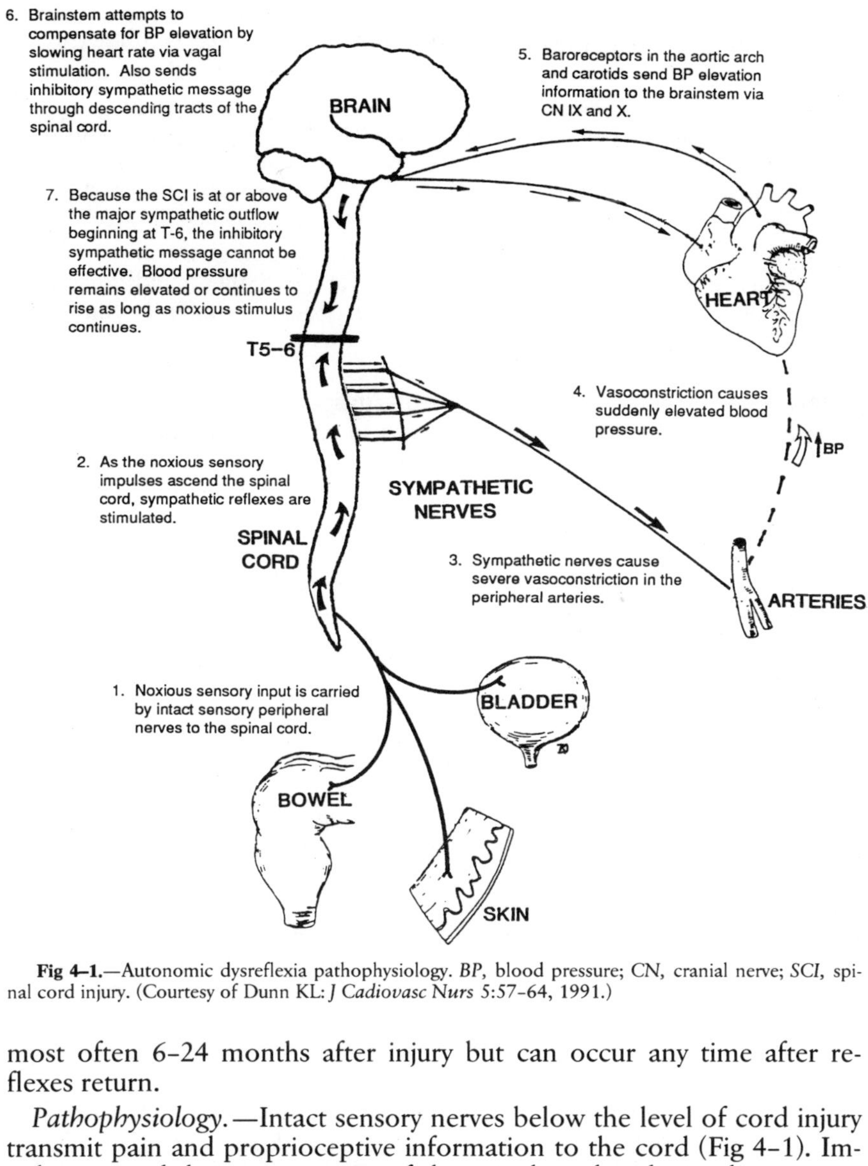

Fig 4–1.—Autonomic dysreflexia pathophysiology. *BP,* blood pressure; *CN,* cranial nerve; *SCI,* spinal cord injury. (Courtesy of Dunn KL: *J Cadiovasc Nurs* 5:57–64, 1991.)

most often 6–24 months after injury but can occur any time after reflexes return.

Pathophysiology.—Intact sensory nerves below the level of cord injury transmit pain and proprioceptive information to the cord (Fig 4–1). Impulses ascend the sensory traits of the spinal cord and stimulate sympathetic neurons in the intermediolateral gray matter columns. The spinal cord injury usually renders the patient unaware of the painful sensations. The sympathetic nerves exit the cord and produce peripheral vasoconstriction by releasing norepinephrine and dopamine from the adrenergic nerve terminals. The cord-injured person is hypersensitive to catecholamines. Disruption of descending inhibitory paths in the spinal cord prevents vasodilation.

Nursing Assessment.—Any noxious sensory input from below the level of the cord injury can trigger AD. Patients tend to have sudden throbbing bitemporal headache, profuse sweating above the lesions, and elevated blood pressure. Patchy erythema may be noted above the level of injury, and pallor may be noted below the level of injury. Other findings may include mydriasis, nasal congestion, cardiac irregularity, and atrioventricular conduction abnormality. Only 10% of patients had bradycardia. A feeling of marked anxiety or impending doom is usual.

Nursing Intervention.—If measures such as elevating the head of the bed and lowering the legs are unavailing, nifedipine may be administered sublingually or orally to control the blood pressure. An indwelling urinary catheter should be checked and cautiously irrigated. The bowel is assessed, checking for stool impaction. Intravenous antihypertensive therapy must be carefully monitored and titrated.

Patient Teaching.—Good bladder and bowel care should be emphasized. Avoiding falls and other injury and the use of proper clothing and shoes can prevent many episodes of AD. Patients should be able to identify episodes at an early stage.

Comments: Sudden, intense headaches, profuse diaphoresis, and hypertension are not the usual assessment findings expected from persons who are quadriplegic. This response, however, is the only way the spinal cord-injured body has "of getting the attention of those around the quadriplegic" to help inactivate the cause the symptoms. The body's compensatory mechanisms are incredibly creative in attempting to protect the individual from harm, even when the normal communication link of the spinal cord is impaired.

Nurse caring for the quadriplegic person has 2 important roles to fulfill. In the first role as care giver, the nurse must anticipate AD by securing PRN orders *before* it develops. Autonomic dysreflexia can occur at any time after reflex activity returns (i.e., 3–6 weeks postinjury). Thus, the nurse working in the critical care, medical-surgical, or rehabilitation unit must be able to recognize and treat AD. Once AD is recognized, the nurse *cannot* wait to page a physician for orders. Action must be taken immediately to determine the cause of the AD and to relieve it. The bladder is the cause of 90% of AD episodes (e.g., bladder distention, bladder spasms, bladder stones, epididymitis, or sphincter/bladder dyssynergia). Other causes include bowel distention, gastrointestinal pathologies (i.e., esophageal reflux), pressures sores, deep vein thrombosis, heterotrophic ossification and fractures.

The second role of the nurse is that of teacher. Family members and the quadriplegic person must be taught by the nurse how to prevent, recognize, and treat AD because it may occur at any time in the patient's lifetime. In addition, quadriplegic persons must be able to teach another person such as an attendant how to recognize and treat AD if it should occur when family members are not present. Although quadriplegic persons are physically unable to correct the problem, they can direct the care given to prevent the problem (preventing a clogged urinary catheter, constipation, and pressure sores) and to treat the problem when it occurs.—S.F. Wilson, RN, PhD

The Effectiveness of Different Methods of Defining Traumatic Brain Injury in Predicting Postdischarge Adjustment in Spinal Cord Injury Population

Richards JS, Osuna FJ, Jaworski TM, Novack TA, Leli DA, Boll TJ (Univ of Alabama, Birmingham)

Arch Phys Med Rehabil 72:275–279, 1991 4–4

Problem.—Severe spinal cord injury (SCI) may also produce concomitant traumatic brain injury (TBI). A prospective investigation was conducted to determine the additional impact of TBI on the overall adjustment of persons with SCI and TBI.

Methods.—A comprehensive, motor-free neuropsychological battery was administered 7 weeks after SCI to 150 patients admitted to a regional SCI center for initial rehabilitation. All patients were at least 16 years of age, and none had a history of psychiatric illness or head injury. Twenty-one patients identified as having SCI and TBI and 21 neurologically matched patients identified as having SCI only were asked to participate with their significant others in a study assessing their long-term adjustment to SCI. Selection criteria for the SCI/TBI and the SCI-only groups included Halstead Category cutoff scores, presence or absence of loss of consciousness, and clinicians' ratings of the severity of TBI. Three trained clinical neuropsychologists who were given all the data and test results served as raters.

Findings.—When the most stringent grouping criteria were used, (all 3 raters in agreement on the presence or absence of TBI), a number of differences emerged for the patient data but not for the significant-other data. Patients who all 3 raters agreed had incurred a concomitant TBI demonstrated greater adjustment difficulty across a variety of measures of personal and family adjustment than did patients who all 3 raters agreed had not incurred a concomitant TBI. However, the 3 raters agreed on whether a TBI had occurred for only 29% of the patients. Consequently, the sample size was too small for meaningful statistical analysis, and only a trend could be identified. Loss of consciousness at the time of injury and lack of agreement in clinical ratings about the presence or absence of TBI were poor predictors of postdischarge adjustment. The TBI severity ratings in the moderate-to-severe range and Halstead Category cutoff scores obtained during initial rehabilitation had some predictive value for postdischarge adjustment in that the more impaired patients with TBI were more likely to have adjustment difficulties as perceived and reported by their significant others than were those with mild TBI.

Conclusion.—These findings underscore the difficulty of making definitive diagnoses of TBI in SCI patients.

Comments: Be alert for spinal cord-injured patients who seem forgetful or agitated. These patients may have experienced a mild TBI at the time of the

SCI. The authors of this article attempted to determine methods to define brain injury in a small sample of patients. Of the 21 TBI patients, the 3 neuropsychologists could agree on the occurrence of TBI in only 6. Those 6 did have greater adjustment difficulty after injury than a matched group of SCI-only patients. Often, TBI is undiagnosed or undetectable. The health care team may not recognize any differences in the patient's personality because they are not acquainted with the patient. Ask the family whether they notice any changes in the patient's behavior or personality. These folks are in the best position to compare. Behavior change may be the first sign of TBI and should be reported. Interestingly, the opposite scenario also can occur. Patients who are admitted with a closed head injury might be found to have a spinal cord injury also when they awake from coma.—S.F. Wilson, RN, PhD

Locked-In Syndrome: A Team Approach

Mauss-Clum N, Cole M, McCort T, Eifler D (VA Med Ctr Palo Alto, Calif; VA Med Ctr Martinsburg, WV)

J Neurosci Nurs 23:273–286, 1991 4–5

Problem.—Locked-in syndrome (LIS) is a condition of brain-stem infarction resulting in quadriplegia, lower cranial nerve paralysis, and mutism with intact cortical function. Such patients remain aware of their internal and external environment, but cannot move or communicate in any way. A team approach to caring for patients with LIS was developed.

Description.—Infarction of the ventral pons, caused by occlusion of the basilar artery, is the most common cause of LIS. The dorsal pons contains structures controlling consciousness and sensation and receives its arterial supply from a network of vessels originating from the basilar and vertebral arteries (Fig 4–2). The exact manifestations depend on the arteries involved and the extent of infarction. In 1 survey, about two thirds of patients were men with a mean age of 52 years. About half of patients had premonitory symptoms, and many had hypertension. The mortality rate was about 60%, and most patients died within 4 months; there was a poor chance for significant recovery.

Nursing Implications.—The nurse's role in the multidisciplinary approach to patients with LIS starts with ensuring a patent airway and monitoring for early neurologic changes. The patient cannot use any available call device, so monitors with alarms must serve as distress signals. Plans are made for pulmonary care and neurologic monitoring, and then comprehensive care is developed more fully. Nursing diagnoses include ineffective airway clearance, impaired verbal communication, anxiety, high risk of thrombophlebitis, activity intolerance, urge incontinence, altered renal function, and high risk of impaired skin integrity. The speech pathologist can assist in facilitating a system of communication; a yes-no response system is vital. Eye blinks may be ineffective because of fatigue and confusion; instead, eyelid closure can be used for

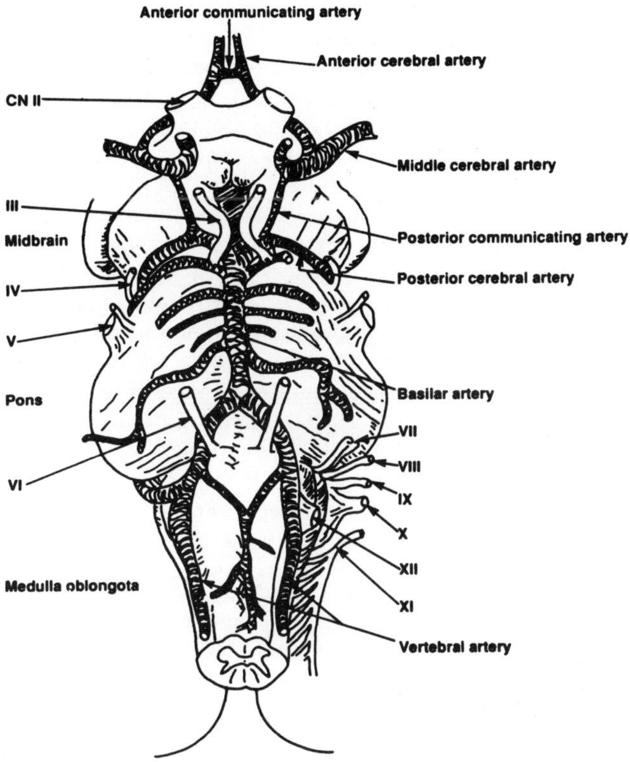

Fig 4–2.—Brain-stem structures and arterial circulation. (Courtesy of Mauss-Clum N, Cole M, McCort T, et al: *J Neurosci Nurs* 23:273–286, 1991.)

no and wide eye opening for yes. A personal communication system must be designed, using an alphabet system or possibly Morse code.

Conclusion.—For all patients with LIS, the treatment plan must be aggressive for the first 4 months after the onset of symptoms. Provision of comprehensive care requires a multidisciplinary approach.

Comments: This syndrome accurately describes the patient's pathology—a mind locked inside a body. These individuals are not only ventilator-dependent quadriplegics because of interruption of the corticospinal tract within the ventral pons, but are also mute with facial and tongue paralysis and dysphagia because of interruption of the cranial nerves that emerge from the brain stem. The description of these patients reminds me of caring for patients with amyotrophic lateral sclerosis (ALS) when their only movement is eye blinking and they are totally aware of what is happening to them.

Communication is a challenge and can be frustrating for everyone involved. The nurses assist patients with their anxiety and frustration without being able to talk with them. Commonly used methods for coping with frustration are verbal (yelling, using profanity) or physical (throwing or hitting something). These individuals can do neither. Allowing the patients to make decisions about their daily routine is helpful in giving them some control over their lives. Talking with the families provides baseline information about the patient's likes and dislikes, previous interests, and coping patterns. These data help in anticipating needs, establishing a plan of care, and creating useful communication techniques. Computerized augmentative communication systems described in this article offer great potential for voluntary expression but require individualization of equipment and software. Continuity in communication and care is enhanced when the same group of nurses care for these patients and their families. These nurses, however, frequently need support from peers to verbalize their own frustrations. I have witnessed nurses who were so frustrated trying to care for and communicate with such patients, that they coped with their frustration by medicating the patient with a PRN drug such as Pavulon and Valium even when the patient did not require it. This action was not harmful to the patient, but it was an intervention that was not therapeutic in resolving the real problem.

Of particular importance is the patient's communication of their preference for resuscitation. Determining the competence of noncommunicating persons presents obvious difficulties. The patient's preference must be determined after medical stability has been accomplished. The 3 patients described in this article all refused the option of cardiopulmonary resuscitation (CPR). When asked about their preference for treatment with antibiotics, all patients requested their use. Even when patients have living wills, we must verify that they still want to abide by the terms of their earlier decisions. In an article by Silverstein et al. (Abstract 13–5), 38 persons with (ALS) were asked about their wishes on life-sustaining therapy. Some of the patients changed their minds from *not wanting* resuscitation to *wanting* resuscitation over a 6-month period.

Refusing the option of CPR means no cardiopulmonary resuscitation but it does not mean withdrawing all life-sustaining treatment! A few months ago, I observed physicians writing orders to withdraw care from patients who signed a do not resuscitate (DNR) consent. The rationale that these physicians gave for writing orders to withdraw care was that "DNR patients do not belong in critical care units. We need to wean them off these drugs and transfer them out of this unit." These physicians were wrong in their interpretation of the DNR consent.

Some patients with LIS do experience some recovery after 12 weeks, with continued improvements over the years. Those with the best prognosis are young, nonhypertensive persons who had a history of vertebrobasilar insufficiency. The recovery is thought to be the result of collateral circulation or resolution of edema from the infarct. Those LIS patients who do not survive deserve a peaceful, comfortable death with dignity.—S.F. Wilson, RN, PhD

The Value of Serial Leg Measurements for Monitoring Deep Vein Thrombosis in Spinal Cord Injury

Swarczinski C, Dijkers M (Rehabilitation Inst of Michigan, Detroit)

J Neurosci Nurs 23:306–314, 1991 4–6

Problem.—Spinal cord injury (SCI) is often complicated by deep vein thrombosis (DVT). Many specialized SCI nursing units use serial leg measures to establish a clinical diagnosis of DVT, although extensive research has shown that the specificity and sensitivity of the clinical signs and symptoms of DVT are not reliable.

Methods.—Daily serial calf and thigh measurements were obtained for 30 patients who spent 920 days in an SCI intensive care unit. Radiofibrinogen uptake tests (RFUTs) were performed about every third day. The 3 criteria for clinical diagnosis of DVT were an increase in calf or thigh circumference from baseline, from the previous day, or a right-left difference of a certain minimal size (more than .5 inch, more than 1 cm, or 1.2 cm and over for women and 1.5 cm and over for men).

Findings.—Such changes and differences correlated only weakly or not at all with RFUT results. Increases and right-left differences considered to be symptomatic occurred very often when no thrombus was found. Variability in these measures and their lack of sensitivity could result from premorbid leg asymmetry, leg atrophy after SCI, changes in circumference caused by factors other than DVT, and a lack of measurement reliability.

Conclusion.—Obtaining serial leg measures is not of value in the diagnosis of DVT in patients with SCI. For those who are reluctant to abandon this practice, the quality of measuring and related decision-making must be improved. More research is needed in this area.

Comments: In my first position as a staff nurse in a rehabilitation hospital, I learned to measure the thigh circumferences of persons with spinal cord injuries. The nurses measured 8 inches above the patella and marked the site of measurement with a marker to ensure that subsequent measurements would be made at the same location. The rationale for this intervention was that swelling of the thigh resulting from DVT could be detected. Pain and Homan's signs were of no use because the patient had no sensation. Redness and heat are other signs that could be used to detect DVT, although they are subjective. Also, redness is difficult to detect in the black population. We were able to identify DVT by the leg measurement method.

This article provides strong evidence that the practice is of questionable use and represents another time-honored nursing ritual refuted by research. Clearly this study needs replication with a larger sample and/or at several sites. How big a problem is DVT in spinal cord-injured persons? In this study of the 30 patients, 14 developed DVT. The incidence reported in the literature varies depending on the diagnostic method used. With clinical criteria, the incidence ranges from 14% to 40%; with impedance plethysmography or venography, it is around 61%; with radiofibrinogen uptake test (RFUT), it is from 70%–100%.

One of the limitations of this study and of thigh measurements in clinical practice is the consistency of measurement needed. A measuring tape that does not stretch must be used. The tape must be placed at the same site on the thigh or calf and be pulled with the same degree of tension each time a measurement is made.

If early detection does not work, there is always prevention. Prevention of DVT is accomplished by use of elastic stockings to increase venous return, adequate hydration to reduce blood viscosity, and range of motion to prevent the lodging of a clot. Aspirin may be helpful in reducing platelet aggregation. Each of these interventions warrants further research to determine its effects on preventing DVT.—S.F. Wilson, RN, PhD

Postocclusive Reactive Hyperemia and Thermal Response in the Skin Microcirculation of Subjects With Spinal Cord Injury

Schubert V, Fagrell B (Huddings Hospital; Karolinska Hospital, Stockholm)
Scand J Rehabil Med 23:33–40, 1991 4–7

Problem.—The sacral area is the most susceptible area for pressure sores in patients with spinal cord injury (SCI). Although the risk of pressure sores is highest just after injury, the risk remains for the rest of the patient's life and seems to increase with age. The external pressure over bony prominences reduces skin blood flow, which leads to ischemia and

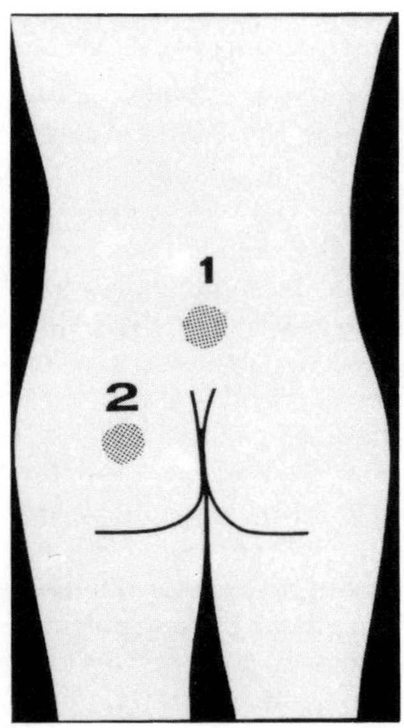

Fig 4–3.—Schematic picture of the 2 measuring points over the sacrum (*1*) and the gluteus maximus muscle (*2*) areas. (Courtesy of Schubert V, Fagrell B: *Scand J Rehabil Med* 23:33–40, 1991.)

tissue damage. Whether the impaired autonomic nerve function in SCI may contribute to a disturbed local microvascular reactivity, resulting in pressure sores in the sacral area, was studied.

Study Methods.—Ten patients with tetraplegia, 10 with paraplegia, and 10 healthy subjects were studied. The patients with SCI were further divided into groups with (N=8) and without (N=12) sensation over the sacral area. Pressure was applied to the skin over the sacrum, then to the gluteus maximus. The movement of blood cells within the area of pressure was measured with the laser Doppler fluxmetry probe, providing data about the skin blood cell flux (SBF) over the sacrum and gluteus maximus muscle (Fig 4–3). The measurements were begun by recording the blood flow without pressure; then pressure was successively increased until there was no blood flow under the probe. To abolish blood flow in the area and cause ischemia in all subjects, a local pressure of 400 mm Hg was needed. Next, the time for blood to return to prepressure flow rates was measured, providing the peak postocclusive hyperemia response.

Findings.—Skin blood flow over the sacrum without applied pressure showed greater values among patients with SCI compared with healthy controls. Also, for SCI patients, SBF occlusion was reached at a lower external skin pressure over the sacrum than over the gluteus maximus. Patients with SCI took longer than healthy subjects to return to the peak blood flow after occlusion in the sacrum, but not in the gluteus maximus. The patients without sensation over the sacrum had a prolonged time to peak SBF over the sacrum than did patients with sensation and healthy persons. The increase of the SBF during postocclusive hyperemia response was lower over the sacrum and gluteus maximus muscle regions in the SCI patients. Temperature responses were weaker in the injured groups than in the healthy group, especially in patients without sensation over the sacrum.

Conclusions.—The reactivity of the skin's microcirculation to locally applied pressure is significantly impaired in patients with SCI. Patients without sensation over the sacrum appear especially to have a disturbed local microvascular reactivity. These microcirculatory and thermal disturbances are probably the result of an impaired autonomic nerve function and may contribute to the high number of pressure sores that occur over the sacral area in SCI patients.

Comments: Skin integrity of individuals with SCI is maintained by turning or use of a special bed or mattress. The ritual for turning is every 2 hours. This is used for any patient who is confined to bed, not just for those with SCI. Our practice should be critically analyzed based on this study, even though the sample size is small. The findings of this study provide a guide for individualizing the turning ritual. Because less pressure is required to occlude the skin blood flow of SCI individuals compared with healthy persons, and because blood flow over the sacrum is slower to return after SCI, SCI persons need more frequent position adjustments.

When individuals with SCI are turned from a supine position, the sacrum must be assessed for color; that is, redness or blanching. If either of these are noted, they should be timed to determine when they disappear. If they do not disappear within 28 minutes ($\pm$18 min) for paraplegics or $\pm$35 minutes to $\pm$23 min for quadriplegics, then we can conclude that the time they stayed supine was too long to provide adequate skin blood flow to the sacrum. These times (28 and 35 minutes) were the times required for blood flow to return to the sacrum after pressure was applied. Also worth noting is that the time required for persons without sensation was longer than for those SCI persons with sensation. Nurses in critical care can apply this knowledge in their practice and can teach it to SCI individuals and family members who will be responsible for the turning after discharge.

The findings of this study do not speak to the value of special beds or mattresses. Although the use of special beds may alter the time allowed in the supine position, the cost of these beds may make their long-term use impractical from an economic viewpoint. Clearly this study needs replication, but it does provide us with important fundamental knowledge on which to base practice to prevent sacral ischemia. Future research studies need to address how much pressure is exerted on the sacrum or other dependent areas to determine the extent to which skin blood flow is impaired.—S.F. Wilson, RN, PhD

Myasthenia Gravis: The Patient in Crisis

Chipps E (Ohio State Univ Columbus)

Crit Care Nurs 11:18–26, 1991 4–8

Pathophysiology.—Myasthenia gravis now is recognized as an autoimmune disorder involving the postsynaptic membrane at the neuromuscular junction. Acetylcholine receptors are markedly reduced, presumably because of an antiacetylcholine receptor antibody. The reduced number of receptor sites results in diminished muscle contraction. The antibody may result from infectious or neoplastic inflammation within the thymus.

Clinical Signs and Symptoms.—Intermittent double vision and eyelid ptosis are early signs of myasthenia gravis. Facial weakness and trouble chewing, swallowing, and speaking occur subsequently, followed by weakness of the neck and extremities. Patients may report trouble climbing stairs and difficulty in daily activities progressing throughout the day. In severe cases, difficulty swallowing increases the risk of aspiration pneumonia. Compromised diaphragm and intercostal muscles may diminish respirations.

Therapeutic Plan.—Anticholinesterase agents are used both diagnostically and therapeutically. Removal of the thymus is always a consideration; thymectomy reportedly leads to remission in half of patients and improvement in many others. Other treatment options include steroids, plasmapheresis, and cytotoxic drugs.

Myasthenic and Cholinergic Crises.—A critical situation may arise from either myasthenic crisis caused by insufficient acetylcholine, often from undermedication, or cholinergic crisis caused by excessive acetylcholine from overmedication. The symptoms of these 2 states are, paradoxically, quite similar.

Nursing Implications.—Frequent assessments of neurologic function, muscle weakness, and respiratory status are essential. Nursing diagnoses include ineffective breathing patterns; ineffective airway clearance; and activity intolerance, all related to severe muscle weakness. Management consists of prompt recognition of the cause of the symptoms and requisite alterations in medications. Should respiratory insufficiency continue, ventilatory support may be required. Symptoms often improve with adequate rest. If tube feeding is inadequate, intravenous hyperalimentation may be necessary to maintain nutritional status.

Comments: Patients with myasthenia gravis are seen in critical care units either because of impending respiratory failure caused by diaphragm or intercostal muscle weakness or because of aspiration pneumonia with or without adult respiratory distress syndrome (ARDS) resulting from pharyngeal weakness. In caring for these patients with respiratory failure, critical care nurses measure or monitor tidal volume and/or vital capacity measurements frequently to determine how much air is moving in and out of the lungs. As the patient's tidal volume approaches <5 to 8 mL/kg body weight, he or she should be evaluated for endotracheal intubation and mechanical ventilation. As the muscle weakness becomes more pronounced, the muscles of respiration are no longer able to provide adequate ventilation.

In caring for any patient with myasthenia gravis, remember that they regain strength after rest. Pace their activities to allow periods of rest between turning, range of motion, bathing, and visiting.

The nurse plays a major role in assessing these patients to determine presence of myasthenic crisis or cholinergic crisis. Often the symptoms are similar, making it difficulty to distinguish and treat the problem. The Tensilon (edrophonium) test is used to distinguish between myasthenic and cholinergic crises. Edrophonium is given (2–10 mg) intravenously. It acts quickly to prevent acetylcholinesterase (AChe) from destroying (hydrolyzing) the acetylcholine (ACh). This allows ACh to interact longer with the ACh receptors sites so that the muscle strength is greater. The Tensilon acts rapidly so that either the symptoms of myasthenia crisis subside or the symptoms of cholinergic crisis become worse. Either way the test determines the cause of the crisis so that it can be treated appropriately. If cholinergic crisis is the cause, atropine is given to reverse the effects of the Tensilon quickly and relieve the symptoms. Appropriate adjustments in anticholinesterase drugs must then be made to prevent recurrence of either crisis.—S.F. Wilson, RN, PhD

A Passage Through Paralysis

Morgan SP (Southwest Florida Regional Med Ctr, Ft Myers)

Am J Nurs 91:70–74, 1991 4–9

Problem.—Guillain-Barré syndrome (GBS) can affect all ages and both sexes worldwide and in any season. It usually starts with a mild upper respiratory infection, followed by an evolving, symmetrical weakness that may begin in the legs and often progresses upward. The course, cause, treatment, and means to assist the patient with GBS were reviewed.

Course and Treatment.—Patients usually progress to complete motor paralysis within a few days, and the muscles do not atrophy until later. Severity depends on the involved nerves; sensory loss is variable, and muscle tenderness and paresthesias are common. Autonomic disturbances usually last no longer than 2 weeks. The respiratory muscles are paralyzed in about 25% of patients. The condition is almost always reversible, plateauing after 2–3 weeks; a shorter plateau period makes long-term disability unlikely. Recovery takes months, often 1 year or longer; 5% of patients die. Treatment is essentially supportive, although plasmapheresis has shortened the acute stage in patients with severe disease. Intravenously administered steroids do not appear to affect the course or prognosis. High-dose intravenously administered gamma globulin is still under study.

Cause.—The cause of the condition is unknown; there does not seem to be any viral invasion of the nervous system. The disease may affect any point of the peripheral nervous system from the nerve root to the distal ending. Inflammatory cells may attack the myelin sheath, resulting in demyelination, inflammation, edema, and nerve compression; the main pathologic finding is segmental demyelination (Fig 4–4). The diagnosis

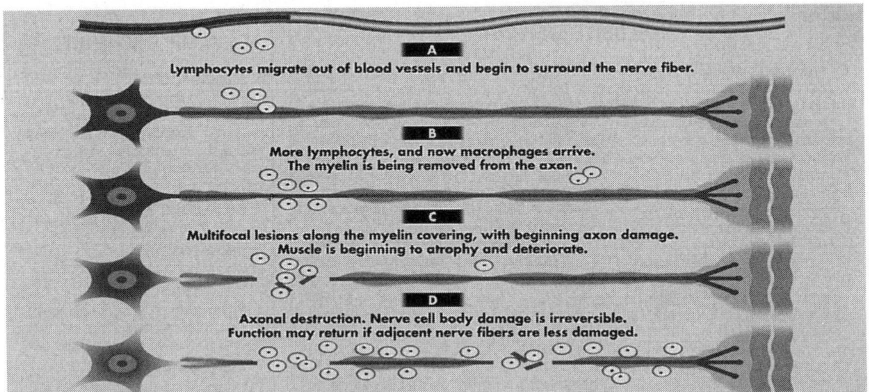

Fig 4–4.—Destructive events in the GBS deterioration phase. (Courtesy of Morgan SP: *Am J Nurs* 91:70–74, 1991.)

may be confirmed by electrophysiologic studies, but the results may be normal if performed early in the course of the disease.

Nursing Considerations.—Respiratory function must be monitored frequently, every 6 hours or more often if respiratory crisis is pending. Assisted ventilation may be started if vital capacity decreases to less than 15 mL/kg. Every 2 hours, the nurse must ask the patient to take a deep breath and slowly count as high as possible and watch for signs of breathlessness, which may indicate grossly reduced ventilatory function. Paresthesias may respond to medications, heat or cold, transcutaneous electrical nerve stimulating, or repositioning. Bladder and bowel function are carefully monitored. A daily bowel regimen is essential in most patients. Communication, such as by an eyeblink system, is a must for intubated, paralyzed patients. Anxiety may be lessened by educating the patient about the disease, its prognosis, treatment, and therapy.

Comment: *See comment after Abstract 4–10.*

Residual Signs in Severe Guillain-Barré Syndrome: Analysis of 57 Patients

de Jager AEJ, Minderhoud JM (University Hospital, Groningen, The Netherlands)

J Neurol Sci 104:151–156, 1991 4–10

Problem.—In patients with acute Guillain-Barré syndrome (GBS), the severity of the axonal damage and paresis are associated with the number of residual signs.

Methods.—To assess the residual signs and social effects of their illness, 57 patients with GBS, with a median age of 38 years, were followed for 2–24 years. All were severely paralyzed and required ventilatory support. During follow-up, 10 patients died, but knowledge of the extent of recovery and social effects of the disease for all patients was obtained either by examination or questionnaire.

Findings.—At follow-up, 35% of patients had recovered completely, 35% had minimal residual motor signs, and 30% had moderate to severe paresis. The most severe residual signs were noted distally in the legs, with the most severe deficits found in muscles innervated by nerves running along an entrapment site. In 49% of patients there were sensory signs, and 58% considered themselves cured; 60% of patients resumed employment, 25% took a less demanding job, and 15% did not return to work. There were significant correlations between degree of residual deficit and severity of weakness in the acute phase and duration of the plateau phase (i.e., artificial ventilation).

Conclusion.—Prognostic factors for patients with GBS are the severity of paresis in the acute phase and the duration of the plateau phase, which is correlated with the length of time on ventilation. Patients with a plateau phase longer than 10 days always had residual signs. As axonal regeneration is slow and often incomplete. The amount of damage in the acute phase determines the duration and outcome of the disease. Motor conduction studies in the acute phase of GBS may help to predict outcome.

Comments: The information from these two articles (Abstracts 4–9 and 4–10) is useful to critical care nurses in teaching patients and families about Guillain-Barré syndrome. The first abstract describes the disease process and the second provides follow-up data on 57 patients who had Guillain-Barré.

Recovery from Guillain-Barré syndrome may or may not be complete. Follow-up studies of patients have found that the amount of damage to the axon in the acute phase determines the duration and outcome of the disease. The acute phase lasts 2–3 weeks followed by a plateau phase recovery that may require months. Patients are responding well to plasmapheresis, which removes the immunoglobulins responsible for the inflammatory response of the peripheral nerves. Nursing diagnoses for these patient may include impaired physical mobility related to muscle weakness, altered breathing pattern related to weak intercostal muscles, and anxiety related to uncertain future.

The follow-up data on patients are important to have when anticipating patient outcomes and when talking with patients and families about prognosis. Most patients recover, and many have no residual motor deficits. Thus, critical care nurses can make a difference in the patient's outcome by preventing complications of bedrest and mechanical ventilation and by ensuring adequate nutrition during the acute process when nerve regeneration begins. These patients commonly experience autonomic nervous system dysfunction manifested by sinus tachycardia, bradycardia, hypertension, orthostatic hypotension, and disturbances of the urinary sphincter. Respiratory complications may occur rapidly and can be identified early by tidal volume and vital capacity measurements.—S.F. Wilson, RN, PhD

Health Education for Self-Management by People With Epilepsy

Legion V (Northwestern Univ, Evanston, Ill)

J Neurosci Nurs 23:300–305, 1991 4–11

Problem.—For patients with epilepsy, behavioral approaches to self-management of seizure control are often obscured by pharmacologic and surgical approaches. Many patients who would benefit from teaching about monitoring and regulating behaviors that affect their susceptibility to seizures never learn about these approaches. The realities and myths about epilepsy and a self-management program were reviewed.

Realities and Myths.—Epilepsy affects 2-4 million children and adults in the United States. It costs Americans more than $3 billion per year in unemployment, underemployment, medical care, premature death, services, and research. Drug treatment can control seizures in about half of patients and can partially control them in 30%. Patients with uncontrolled disease are confronted with fear and uncertainty. In 1 study, more than 75% of patients reported depression; about 20% thought about suicide; almost 25% frequently wished they were dead. The social stigma of the condition has negative consequences.

Behavioral Approach.—In a holistic view of epilepsy, seizures result from a chain of events between affected people and their environments. It is important to ask how the patient's seizure-free days differ from those in which he or she has a seizure. Most epileptic patients report that emotional stress brings on their seizures, and many can predict which events will cause seizures. Others report that deviation from healthy practices, such as rest, diet, and drug treatment, bring on seizures. A comprehensive self-management program for newly diagnosed patients includes confronting the associated myths and stigma, reviewing the diagnostic procedures, and discussing the psychological problems and coping mechanisms. Patients are given a realistic evaluation of their risks and are taught to identify and watch for precipitating factors. The most important behavioral technique is progressive relaxation and other stress management methods. Patients need information on insurance, driving, and work; on sex and reproduction; and the effects on family life. They must know how to use their medications and how to identify and resolve their feelings about their disease.

Conclusion.—Behavioral self-management can help psychosocial adjustment and the effectiveness of medical treatment for epilepsy. Such training should be considered a key part of epilepsy treatment.

Comments: This article contains 2 important points for the critical care nurse. The first is the use of the mind-body connection to reduce seizures in epiletics. Our care includes administering anticonvulsant drugs and teaching the patient and family about these drugs, their side effects, how to prevent seizures, and how to care for the person during a seizure. A holistic view of the person with epilepsy also reveals the effects of stress, both personal and environmental, on the incidence of seizures. To address these issues, we must include, as a part of our teaching, the importance of progressive relaxation and other stress management techniques. Equally important are practices of a healthy diet and adequate rest. After teaching these patients about relaxation and guiding them in a relaxation session, have them identify when and where they could practice relaxation so that it can become a part of their daily behavior. Consider what other patient populations would benefit from relaxation therapy. Relaxation has been used to lower heart rate and blood pressure.

The second point of this article is the source of the information: the patients. When we care for patients who have chronic health problems we can obtain valuable information by asking them how this chronic condition has affected their lives, what adaptations they have made, and how we might change our teaching to help others adapt to disease. Patients can be very creative in their adaptations to chronic illness. Their adaptations can be shared with others. Based on their feedback, we also may find the need to adjust our patient teaching to make it more useful. The education about how to live with disease should be a 2-way exchange. We can learn a great deal about how to live with illness from our patients.—S.F. Wilson, RN, PhD

Status Epilepticus: Clinical Features, Pathophysiology, and Treatment

Watson C (Univ of California, Davis)

West J Med 155:626–631, 1991 4–12

Introduction.—Status epilepticus is a state of continuing or recurring seizures, remitting incompletely between attacks. Any type of seizure can occur in status form (Table 1). An estimated 60,000 episodes of tonic-clonic status epilepticus occur in the United States each year. Children are affected most often, but status epilepticus also is frequent in those older than 60 years. Many episodes occur after acute insult or injury, whether or not there is a history of epilepsy or another neurologic disorder.

Management.—The pathophysiologic factors in status epilepticus are shown in Fig 4–5. Comprehensive evaluation of the patient (Table 2) is the critical first step, specifically seeking evidence of focal neurologic signs, head trauma, and CNS infection. Phenytoin is effective in controlling seizures and has a relatively long half-life. It does not cause significant CNS depression. One approach is to control seizures rapidly with a benzodiazepine and then to administer phenytoin for its sustained anti-epileptic action. Phenobarbital also has a long half-life and is effective against both generalized and focal seizures, but it tends to depress consciousness and may contribute to respiratory depression.

Comments: I was thrilled when I read this article because recently I assisted a student caring for a patient in the intensive care unit who had status epilepticus. The treatment protocol was less than clear and efficient. I copied the tables and figure included here from the article for my student and to add to my notebook containing "Pearls of Wisdom". Because this seizure sequence is not a common occurrence, the nurse needs the protocol close at hand.

Critical care nurses identify status epilepticus and initiate a treatment protocol to minimize the time of seizing to preserve brain function. The brain normally uses 20% of the body's oxygen supply and 25% of the glucose supply. During a seizure, these percentages increase. During the first 30 minutes, the lactate increases, causing acidosis resulting from anaerobic metabolism. This metabolic acidosis then causes constriction of the cerebral vessels, reducing blood flow further. FIgure 4–5 shows the compensation on mechanisms that occur during status epilepticus and approximately when brain damage occurs. Applying the appropriate knowledge and skills, the critical care nurse can make a difference for the patient with status epilepticus.—S.F. Wilson, RN, PhD

TABLE 1.—Classification of Status Epilepticus

Class	Type
Generalized convulsive status epilepticus	Tonic-clonic
	Tonic
	Clonic
	Myoclonic
Generalized nonconvulsive status epilepticus	Absence
Simple partial (focal) status epilepticus	Somatomotor-epilepsia partialis continua
	Sensory-somatosensory, special sensory
	Aphasic
	Autonomic
Complex partial status epilepticus	

(Courtesy of Watson C: *West J Med* 155:626–631, 1991.)

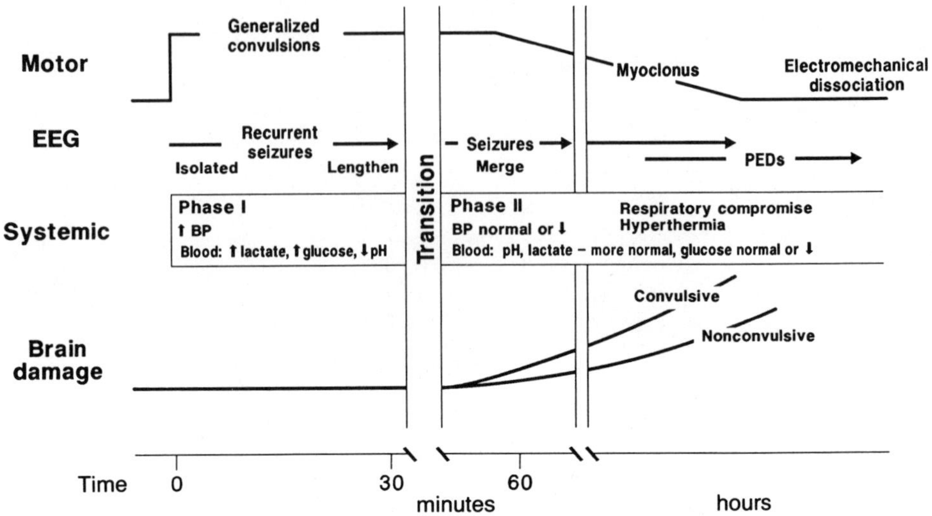

Fig 4–5.—The diagram shows the evolution of pathophysiologic changes during status epilepticus (adapted with permission from Lothman EW: *Neurology* 40 (suppl 2): 13–23, 1990.). *BP,* blood pressure; *PEDS,* periodic epileptiform discharges. (Courtesy of Watson C: *West J Med* 155:626–631, 1991.)

TABLE 2.—Treatment of Status Epilepticus

Time Frame	Procedure
0–5 min	Assess cardiorespiratory function, take history, and perform neurologic and physical examination; draw blood specimens for antiepileptic drug levels, glucose, BUN, creatinine, calcium, magnesium, electrolytes, complete blood count, metabolic screen, drug screen, and arterial blood gases; insert of oral airway and administer oxygen if needed
6–9 min	Start IV infusion with saline solution; administer 25 grams glucose and B vitamins
10–45 min	Infuse lorazepam, 0.1 mg/kg (4 to 8 mg), at <2 mg/min Also begin infusion of phenytoin, 20 mg/kg, at a rate of 25 mg/min; this may take 20 to 40 min; monitor ECG, respirations, and blood pressure If seizures persist, give additional phenytoin, 5 mg/kg, at same rate, and, if needed, another 5 mg/kg until a maximum of 30 mg/kg has been given
40–60 min	If seizures persist, intubate and give phenobarbital, 20 mg/kg, at <100 mg/min IV
1 hour	If seizures persist, pentobarbital coma or general anesthesia should be started

Abbreviations: *BUN*, blood urea nitrogen; *IV*, intravenous.
(Courtesy of Watson C: *West J Med* 155:626–631, 1991.)

5 Altered Metabolism

Hyperadrenergic States

Breslow MJ, Ligier B (Johns Hopkins Med Inst, Baltimore)

Crit Care Med 19:1566–1579, 1991 5–1

Purpose.—Selected conditions in which catecholamines are present in higher than normal concentrations were reviewed. The physiologic and pathophysiologic hyperadrenergic states and the use of sympathomimetic drugs were discussed.

Data Sources.—Pharmacologic and physiologic studies in the literature were reviewed. The research involved animals or humans.

Findings.—A variety of clinical situations are associated with increased levels of plasma catecholamines. After major injury, catecholamines support vital organ perfusion and mobilize fuel substrates. After surgical trauma and during acute diseases, however, catecholamine-induced physiologic changes can interact with underlying disease processes and produce significant complications. (Plasma catecholamines are also raised in patients with pheochromocytoma.) Exogenous catecholamines are used to treat a variety of conditions, such as anaphylaxis and various shock states. The sympathomimetic agents available differ in their ability to stimulate various subpopulations of adrenergic receptors. These differences allow astute clinicians to attain specific physiologic end-points.

Conclusions.—With a knowledge of the pharmacology of sympathomimetic agents and the physiologic consequences of adrenergic receptor stimulation, clinicians can prevent undesirable catecholamine effects and use these drugs to reach therapeutic goals.

Comments: Can you bring to mind the image of stress—what it looks like and feels like? Have you ever wondered about the remarkable compensatory efforts of the body when its physical or emotional integrity has been breached? Why, in times of stress, do neuroendocrinologic processes convene for the purpose of increasing blood glucose levels, blood volume, and cardiac output? There is speculation that such processes are evolutionary adaptations rooted in prehistoric times, times when humans were part of the food chain for large carnivorous reptiles, and trauma was a common malady. Without emergency medical systems and hospitals, endogenous interventions were necessary to maintain circulating blood volume and energy substrate for brain functioning in the presence of trauma. Today, these neuroendocrine responses to stress are less vital and, if excessive, may actually prove detrimental.

This article provides an indepth look at the adrenergic responses to stress as well as adrenergic agonist drugs and conditions in which catecholamines are present in supranormal concentrations (e.g., pheochromocytoma). When epinephrine and norepinephrine, the principle endogenous catecholamines, are released in abundance from the adrenal medulla, heart activity is increased and blood flow is detoured away from less needy areas of the body. Epinephrine, along with other "stress hormones" (cortisol, growth hormone, and glucagon), ensure sufficient energy substrate by increasing blood glucose production, lipolysis, and protein catabolism. To assure sufficient circulating blood volume, antidiuretic hormone and aldosterone work on renal reabsorptive processes. The body's integrated and adaptive response to stress is remarkable and profound. It is beneficial in some instances (e.g., hemorrhagic shock), and damaging in others (e.g., myocardial infarction).

Unfortunately, the body cannot discriminate among stressors, whether they are emotional or physical, associated with trauma or heart failure. For this reason, nurses must be keenly aware of the potential harmful effects of the stress response. This is especially important because many of the sympathomimetic agents we give to critically ill patients (e.g., dopamine, levophed) elicit various effects of the stress response. How can we potentiate the positive effects of stress hormones and ablate the negative? More research is needed. Perhaps it is time to reexamine the value of nontraditional stress reduction techniques within the critical care arena (e.g., relaxation therapy, music therapy, guided imagery)—an area of practice where nurses can have tremendous impact. One thing is for certain. The next time you feel the telltale symptoms of stress, recall the physiologic sequelae of hyperadrenergic function, described in this article, and take immediate steps to "chill out!"— C. Kessler RN, MN, CCRN, CS

Understanding Serum Electrolytes: How to Avoid Mistakes

Kapsner CO, Tzamaloukas AH (Univ of New Mexico, Albuquerque)

Postgrad Med 90:151–161, 1991 5–2

Purpose.—Serum electrolytes must be interpreted in light of the principles of serum electrolyte concentrations; a single value usually cannot be interpreted by itself. These principles are illustrated and recommendations are made based on actual case examples.

Discussion.—Serum sodium provides only an indirect estimate of tonicity. Abnormal sodium concentration usually results from concurrent abnormalities in total body sodium and water. Sodium and water depletion are signaled by orthostatic hypotension and tachycardia, persistent thirst, dry skin and mucous membranes, and low urine flow rate with a high ratio of serum urea to creatinine. A common error is assuming that hyponatremia means decreased total body sodium. The relation of body solute to body water is indicated by serum osmolality. Serum osmolality provides the same information as serum sodium concentration in the absence of excess nonsodium solute. If such an excess is present, osmolality is increased, and this not reflected by an increase in serum sodium concentration. Neither serum sodium concentration nor osmolality is an accurate indicator of serum tonicity when solutes with both body water and extracellular distributions are present.

Acid-base disorder is not excluded by a normal bicarbonate level; it is also a mistake to assume that external potassium balance alone determines serum potassium levels; it is also determined by internal potassium balance. Patients with shifting of cellular potassium into the extracellular compartment may have hyperkalemia even when they have a deficit of total body potassium; those with increased cellular uptake may have hypokalemia even with adequate total body potassium. Patients with acid-base abnormalities may have altered serum chloride concentration, regardless of changes in serum sodium concentration. Patients with an increased anion gap have acid-base abnormalities even when other parameters are normal. The anion gap also may be useful in evaluating metabolic acidosis. The anion gap should be computed even when bicarbonate level is normal.

Conclusions.—The difficulty of interpreting isolated serum electrolyte levels is stressed. Cases and comments illustrating the importance of knowing the principles of serum electrolyte concentrations are presented.

Comments: How often have you or a member of your health care team made decisions about intervention based on an isolated serum electrolyte abnormality and later realized that the intervention was not correct because you did not have adequate information about the patient? Certainly, it is always essential to consider the patient's history, physical assessment, and other laboratory data before making clinical decisions about the management of a specific electrolyte.

This article is particularly helpful in its discussion of frequent errors made in assessing serum sodium, potassium, bicarbonate, chloride, and anion gap data. The most common error made with each electrolyte is highlighted by a short patient example followed by a commentary, which makes the article especially useful to practicing clinicians. The information is invaluable for critical care nurses who continuously collaborate with other members of the health care team in the interpretation of perplexing electrolyte imbalances.—L.E. Lancaster, RN, MSN, EdD

Magnesium Metabolism: A Case Report and Literature Review

Friday BA, Reinhart RA (St Joseph's Hosp, Marshfield, Wis; Marshfield Clinic)

Crit Care Nurse 11:62–72, 1991 5–3

Physiology.—After potassium, magnesium is the most abundant intracellular cation. It is especially active in metabolic reactions contributing to the production and use of adenosine triphosphate (ATP). All enzy-

Clinical Manifestations of Magnesium Deficiency

Cardiac

- Electrocardiographic
  - Premature ventricular complexes
  - T-wave flattening
  - Atrial fibrillation
  - Torsade de pointes
- Coronary artery spasm
- Enhanced sensitivity to digitalis intoxication
- Possible greater size of myocardial infarction
- Possible enhanced susceptibility to ventricular fibrillation and sudden death in ischemic heart disease

Neuromuscular

- Muscle weakness
- Muscle twitching and tremor
- Positive Chvostek's sign
- Delirium
- Hyperreflexia
- Convulsions
- Coma

Metabolic

- Refractory hypokalemia
- Hypocalcemia

(Courtesy of Friday BA, Reinhart RA: *Crit Care Nurse* 5:62–72, 1991.)

matic reactions involving ATP require magnesium ions. Within cells, magnesium ions affect the function of organelles such as the sarcoplasmic reticulum through altering calcium flux. The ion also affects sodium, calcium, and potassium channels in the cell membrane.

Altered Electrolyte Balance.—Hypermagnesemia most often results from renal insufficiency and is most likely if magnesium-containing antacids or laxatives have been used. Hypotension and ECG abnormalities occur at serum levels of 2.5–5.0 mM/L. At higher levels, areflexia and respiratory muscle weakness can develop. Cardiac arrest may occur at levels above 12.5 mM/L. Rhythm disorders may result from a loss of intracellular potassium secondary to hypomagnesemia (table).

Nursing Implications.—A single intravenous dose of magnesium can be effective, but repeated doses are needed to replete intracellular stores. Reversible hypotension can occur when magnesium is given rapidly. Oral supplementaion is generally well tolerated.

Comments: When was the last time you assessed your critically ill patient for a magnesium imbalance. Critical care nurses typically assess for sodium, potassium, and fluid imbalances, but evaluation of magnesium balance is often overlooked in the clinical assessment.

Because the kidneys are important in maintaining magnesium balance, hypermagnesemia is usually related to renal insufficiency and renal failure. Hypomagnesemia is often related to renal losses; however, in critically ill patients it can be related to poor intestinal absorption and prolonged intravenous therapy without magnesium supplementation. Almost every critically ill patient fits into at least one of the etiologic categories that could lead to magnesium imbalances.

This article uses a clinical example of a patient with a malignant ventricular dysrhythmia who responded to magnesium supplementation. The patient problems related to hypomagnesemia highlighted in the clinical example are then discussed from a pathophysiologic standpoint. Although the emphasis is on the effects of hypomagnesemia on the heart, there is adequate discussion of other assessment parameters for magnesium deficiency, especially in relation to the neuromuscular system. The information in the article would assist nurses in assessing for magnesium deficiency in all critically ill patients and in understanding the basis for its pharmacologic management. It could serve as the basis for a continuing education lecture and for preparing a standardized assessment for magnesium imbalances.—L.E. Lancaster, RN, MSN, EdD

Rewarming Postoperative Patients: Lights, Blankets, or Forced Warm Air

Giuffre M, Finnie J, Lynam DA, Smith D (DC Gen Hosp, Washington, DC; Mary Hitchcock Mem Hosp, Hanover, NH; St Elizabeth's, Boston)
J Post Anesth Nurs 6:387–393, 1991 5–4

Problem.—Patients returning from surgery have reduced body temperatures. A study was done to see whether the forced warm air system was more effective than warmed cotton blankets or radiant heat lamps for rewarming patients after surgery.

Study Methods.—Ninety patients were enrolled in the study. Postanesthesia Care Unit (PACU) temperatures in these patients were 95°F or less. The patients were randomly assigned to 1 of 3 intervention groups: warmed cotton blankets, radiant heat lamps, or forced warm air. Oral or axillary temperatures were monitored every 15 minutes. Warming interventions were continued until patients had a temperature of 96.8°F.

Findings.—Mean rewarming times for patients who shivered were comparable in all 3 groups. Among those who did not shiver, the forced warm air treatment rewarmed significantly faster than did the other 2 treatments. Nonshivering patients in the forced warm air group were ready to be discharged somewhat sooner than nonshivering patients in the other 2 groups.

Conclusions.—Warm cotton blankets were recommended for patients who shivered after surgery. Shivering patients seemed to find the blankets conforting. Nonshivering patients receiving forced air therapy rewarmed 63 minutes faster than nonshivering patients treated with radiant heat lamps and 77 minutes faster than those given blankets. Further study is needed to determine the relative comfort provided by these methods.

Comments: Unlike the lizard, humans are homothermous, able to maintain a temperature within a very narrow range through peripheral vascular constriction and heat production from increased muscle tone. However, patients undergoing anesthesia lose their thermoregulatory capabilities and, with exposure to the cool operating room environment, become poikilothermic, or cold blooded, much like our lizard friends. Intraoperative hypothermia is a therapeutic intervention in cardiac surgery to protect the myocardium, decrease metabolism, and provide a bloodless operative field (1). Even in situations where hypothermia is not intentionally induced for surgery, postoperative temperature reductions of 2°–3°C (3.6°–5.4°F) are common. Although intraoperative hypothermia is potentially dangerous (altering drug and anesthetic elimination and causing cardiac and acid-base disturbances), hypothermia persisting into the postoperative recovery period is actually associated with most adverse effects.

What are the safest and most effective rewarming practices? This award-winning study gives the nod to use of forced warm air over the standard practices of warm blankets and radiant heat. Although all of these approaches work, stabilization of body temperature can be reached approximately an hour sooner with forced warm air. Is sooner better? The authors of this article do not answer this question; nor do they make it clear what degree of temperature changes occurred during the rewarming process. It has been recommended that patients be rewarmed no faster than 1°C per hour and that the rewarming activities be focused on the patient's trunk. These precautions would reduce the risk of "rewarming shock," which would occur if the patient's periphery is rewarmed while the core is still cool, causing a rapid displacement of intravascular volume to the periphery and subsequent hypotension (2). The best speed for rewarming and the problem of rewarming shock are issues requiring further study.

More study is also required in the use of forced warm air in rewarming cardiac surgical patients. Like radiant heat, forced warm air decreases peripheral vasoconstriction, a beneficial side effect for cardiac surgical patients who initially maintain high systemic vascular resistance. A related problem is that of hyperthermia, which is frequently manifested within 12 hours of cardiac surgery. Does forced warm air hasten this manifestation?

Summers (3) provides a detailed discussion of hypothermia, both intentional and accidental, and is recommended reading for nurses interested in learning more about "the big chill."—C. Kessler, RN, MN, CCRN, CS

References

1. Howie J: Hypothermia and rewarming after cardiac operation. *Focus on Crit Care,* 18:414–418, 1991.
2. Halloway N: Therapeutic hypothermia, in: Halloway N (ed): *Nursing in the Critically Ill Adult,* Menlo Park, CA, Addison-Wesley, 1984, 355–356.
3. Summers S: Hypothermia: One nursing diagnosis or three? *Nurs Diag* 3:2–11, 1992.

6 Hematology

Heparin-Induced Thrombocytopenia and Thrombosis

Waldrop GB, Cervenka BS, Moffett SA, Bedenbaugh JC, Bishop LB, Crouch MA (Self Mem Hosp, Greenwood, SC; Community Longterm Care, Greenwood)

Dimens Crit Care Nurs 10:330–344, 1991 6–1

Problem.—Heparin-induced thrombocytopenia and thrombosis syndrome (HITTS), also known as white clot syndrome, occurs 2 or more days after initiation of heparin therapy in 1% to 10% of patients receiving heparin. One study of HITTS reported a 21% incidence of limb amputation and a 29% mortality rate. The most widely accepted explanation of the pathophysiology of HITTS is that an immune-mediated response to heparin results in platelet aggregation.

Case Report.—A woman was admitted to the surgical unit with a medical diagnosis of ischemic rest pain of the left foot. Initial medical diagnoses were aortoiliac occlusive disease, hypertension, and chronic obstructive pulmonary disease (COPD) with emphysematous changes. Initial nursing diagnoses were alteration in comfort related to ischemic pain in left foot and anxiety related to hospitalization and anticipated procedures. The patient had HITTS and underwent 2 surgeries for occlusive disease, including a left nephrectomy. The surgeries were ultimately followed by bilateral above-the-knee amputations, increased renal failure, and death. The nursing diagnoses were (1) actual or potential alteration in tissue perfusion related to thrombosis and thrombocytopenia, (2) potential for impaired gas exchange related to ventilation/perfusion mismatch, (3) pain related to impaired tissue perfusion, (4) anxiety or fear related to potential loss of body functions and threat of death, (5) hopelessness related to ramifications of disease process, and (6) knowledge deficit related to disease process and prescribed treatments.

Nursing Management.—Key nursing actions for the early recognition and treatment of patients with HITTS include collaborating with the physician on the definitive diagnosis, discontinuing heparin as soon as HITTS is suspected and assessing for evidence of thrombosis and hemorrhage, preventing thrombotic and hemorrhagic complications, controlling pain, supporting and educating the patient and family, and reevaluating practice standards to limit random use of heparin and to encourage routine monitoring of platelet counts and partial thromboplastin time (PTTs) during heparin therapy.

Nursing Implications.—Because many critical care patients are potentially at risk for HITTS because of exposure to heparin, the nurse's most important role is routine patient assessment for evidence of thromboembolic complications and hemorrhage. Declining platelet counts, increased heparin requirements to maintain a satisfactory PTT, or a new or recurrent thrombosis or hemorrhage should alert the nurse to the possibility of HITTS. Immediate cessation of heparin is essential to reduce morbidity and mortality.

Comment: *See comment after Abstract 6–2.*

Analysis of the Research About Heparinized Versus Nonheparinized Intravascular Lines

Peterson FY, Kirchhoff KT (Boise State Univ, Idaho; Univ of Utah, Salt Lake City)

Heart Lung 20:631–642, 1991 6–2

Problem.—Current practice mandates a flush procedure to maintain patency of vascular catheters and prevent complications, but the practice has been questioned. A change from the use of a heparinized saline solution to a nonheparinized solution has a basis in cost savings and patient well-being. Published and unpublished research on the efficacy of dilute heparin solutions and normal saline solutions in flushing and maintaining the patency of vascular catheters was reviewed and analyzed.

Study Methods.—Following an online and manual literature search covering 1968 through 1990, 20 research reports were coded and analyzed quantitatively and qualitatively. The 20 studies involved both intravenous and intraarterial catheters in pediatric and adult patients. Two were unpublished studies, 1 was a nursing master's thesis, 1 was from a medical journal, 7 were from pharmacy journals, and 9 were from nursing journals. Thirteen conceptually similar studies were subjected to meta-analysis to aggregate and summarize data using an explicit set of analytic rules.

Findings.—The results of the 13 studies used in the meta-analysis were nonsignificant, with no difference in duration of patency between heparin and saline flush solutions. The analysis revealed vast differences in reporting among journals, with a marked lack of statistical analyses reported in most of the clinical nursing journals.

Conclusions.—Meta-analysis of 13 studies revealed no significant difference between heparin and saline flush procedures in peripheral intravenous catheters. This finding is supported quantitatively by the low average effect size and qualitatively by the research data. Saline solution used as a peripheral intravenous flush solution effectively maintained catheter patency, decreased the complications of heparin, and did not significantly increase the incidence of phlebitis. The 1 discrepant study had serious weaknesses. The comparable performance of the 2 flush solutions may provide an alternative to heparin use, thereby reducing patient complications and cost.

Comments: I find it puzzling that nurses are so quick to embrace new technologies yet so reluctant to give up unsubstantiated nursing rituals. That the ritual is of little value seems to raise few eyebrows. Apparently, documentation of serious complications from the ritual is required before reexamination of practice occurs and the nursing ritual is tossed out with discards from the past such as soap suds enemas and mustard plaster. The documented risk of heparin-induced thrombocytopenia and thrombosis syndrome (HITTS), has finally caused us to reexamine the practice of routine heparin flushes to maintain patency of vascular catheters.

Waldrop et al. (Abstract 6–1) use a detailed case study to discuss HITTS, or white clot syndrome. First reported in 1952, this fascinating disorder has been largely ignored, despite the relatively high morbidity and mortality rates associated with the syndrome. This article does an admirable job in describing the pathophysiology and treatment of HITTS. The authors state that immediate cessation of heparin is essential to reduce the risk of lethal thromboembolic events associated with HITTS. They also implore nurses to halt the practice of using heparinized flushes to maintain patency of intermittent intravenous infusion devices. If heparin should not be used, can saline flushes be used with the same efficacy? Happily, the answer is yes. Results of an exhaustive review of the literature and a nationwide nursing survey by Peterson and Kirchhoff (Abstract 6–2) have provided sufficient evidence to propel another nursing ritual into obsolescence. Not only is saline an effective flush for maintaining patency in peripheral intermittent infusion devices, it also causes fewer complications, does not interact with other drugs, and is cost-effective. An estimated annual savings of $10,000 to $66,000 has been reported in some hospitals. The efficacy of saline flushes for maintaining patency in central lines has not yet been substantiated by research. The efficacy of heparinized flush solutions for maintaining arterial catheter patency has been demonstrated, however, by the American Association of Critical-Care Nurses' "Thunder Project" research. (See comments for Abstract 1–4.) Hopes are high that heparin, one of the most frequently prescribed drugs in the United States, will no longer be required for maintaining patency of intravascular lines, thus reducing the threat of HITTS.

We must look at our nursing practice with fresh eyes. Is what we commonly do based on sound research? Does it even work? Is it reasonably cost-effective in this era of the "bottom-line?" If the answer to any of these is "no," then it is time to get rid of meaningless habits and move on. Gosh, maybe it's time to reevaluate those anti-aging creams in my medicine cabinet. . . .—C. Kessler, RN, MN, CCRN, CS

Bedside Diagnostic Blood Testing: Its Accuracy, Rapidity, and Utility in Blood Conservation

Salem M, Chernow B, Burke R, Stacey J, Slogoff M, Sood S (Johns Hopkins Univ, Baltimore; Harvard Med School, Boston)

JAMA 266:382–389, 1991 6–3

Problem.—Traditional biochemical assessment of critically ill patients is time consuming and requires excessive phlebotomy. In addition, the measurements may not always be accurate. It now is possible by using microchemistry instruments to acquire blood test results rapidly and reliably with the use of only drops of whole blood.

Study Methods.—A prospective 1-year study was undertaken at a tertiary acute care teaching hospital and a university-affiliated community hospital to evaluate the use of microchemistry technology (using the NOVA State Profile 5 analyzer). A paired sample comparison study was done to assess the NOVA with reference to standard clinical laboratory instruments. Additionally, whole blood samples were analyzed in the intensive care unit (ICU) setting using the mobile bedside microchemistry instrument. A total of 529 paired blood samples was analyzed for blood gases, electrolytes, and hematocrit.

Findings.—Results obtained by using the microchemistry instrument correlated closely with those yielded by conventional laboratory methods. There was, however, more variability in some analyses when samples were first studied in the ICU by using the microchemistry instrument and then transported to the laboratory for "stat" determinations. Except for sodium, there was a strong correlation ($R > .90$) between blood chemistry determinations when central laboratory instruments or bedside microchemistry instruments were used. Sodium values were slightly (artificially) altered by the amount of anticoagulant (heparin sodium) remaining in the phlebotic syringe.

Nursing Implications.—The use of a multichannel microchemistry instrument in the ICU provides accurate analyses of blood chemical components and provides a significant savings of both time and blood. This approach simplifies the urgent biochemical evaluation of critically ill patients.

Comments: "Stat" blood studies are a crucial element in the management of acutely ill patients. Traditional methods of laboratory analysis of the patient's biochemical status frequently cause critical care nurses to throw up their hands in exasperation. Lengthy turnaround times, the excess phlebotomy of patients, lost laboratory specimens, and the occasional inaccuracy of laboratory measurements can impede vital interventions in the critically ill patient. How can we simplify urgent biochemical assessment of acutely ill patients while limiting iatrogenic blood loss and ensuring accuracy of the results? The answer may be the use of a "bedside laboratory."

Bedside microchemistry technology has been available for more than 5 years but has lacked sufficient evaluation to warrant its use in critical care settings. The ambitious study described in this article makes a convincing pitch for use of this new "portable" technology. Imagine accurate biochemical determinations reported within 2 to 10 minutes! Most hospital central laboratories have a mean turnaround time of more than 1 hour for "stat" determinations of electrolytes and hematocrit. In addition to "time-saving" benefits, there were "blood-saving" benefits as well. The routine "leeching" of critical care patients has been an ignored and barbaric ritual. In 1986, Smoller and Kruskall reviewed the phlebotomy practices within a tertiary hospital and found that critical care patients were phlebotomized a mean of 3.4 times per day, with a total mean volume of 41.5 mL of blood per day. Over the course of their critical care stay, the patient averaged a 762.2-mL blood loss through laboratory phlebotomies. This amount was higher in patients with indwelling arterial lines (1). The microchemistry technology evaluated in the current study by Salem et al. demonstrated a greater than 70% reduction in blood loss when compared with routine laboratory phlebotomy practices.

Bedside microchemistry instrument use does appear to live up to its claims. However, does the increased speed of laboratory determinations actually alter morbidity and mortality the way logic suggests? Because of the need for trained staff to run the "on-unit laboratories" and comply with quality control procedures, is it cost-effective enough to warrant its use in all critical care areas? Can microchemistry technology be effectively translated to central laboratory methods to minimize patient blood loss and maximize accuracy? These questions must be answered before we embrace this new technology. Until then, we must be more prudent in the number and volume of blood draws obtained. It also appears that for now, when ordering "stat" blood draws, we will simply have to "hurry up and wait."—C. Kessler, RN, MN, CCRN, CS

Reference

1. Smoller BR, Kruskall MS: Phlebotomy for diagnostic laboratory tests in adults. *N Engl J Med* 314:1233–1235, 1986.

7 Infection

Prevention of Central Venous Catheter Sepsis: A Prospective Randomized Trial

Bonawitz SC, Hammell EJ, Kirkpatrick JR (Western Pennsylvania Hosp, Pittsburgh)

Am Surg 57:618–623, 1991 7–1

Problem and Purpose.—There is considerable disagreement about the management of central venous catheters (CVCs), including the best timing of catheter exchange to prevent infection. This is a particular problem in the intensive care unit (ICU). The implantable collagen cuff may represent an important step toward preventing catheter infection. A prospective study of the role of routine catheter changes and implantable collagen cuff in reducing the incidence of catheter infection in critically ill patients is reported.

Study Methods.—Over a 14-month study period, 159 CVCs were placed in 85 surgical ICU patients. At study entry, the patients were randomized to 1 of 4 groups; catheters were routinely removed every 3 or 7 days, and the implantable collagen cuff was either used or not used. When catheters were removed, the central line tip, insertion site, and peripheral blood were cultured.

Findings.—Incidence of catheter colonization was 16.4% and incidence of catheter infection was 2.5%. There were no significant differences in catheter colonization rates or infection rates at 3 vs. 7 days. Neither were there any significant differences with regard to the use of the collagen cuff.

Conclusions.—Changing CVCs every 3 days offers no significant advantage over changing them every 7 days in terms of preventing catheter infection. The implantable collagen cuff does not reduce infection rate in critically ill patients who require multiple lumen CVCs.

Comments: How long do we have to ask the same old questions before we get definitive answers? An echoing question examined by the authors of this study is how frequently should CVCs be replaced? Did they find a conclusive answer? No. They did find, however, that replacing central lines every 3 days offered no benefit over catheter exchange every 7 days. Their findings seem to be supported by Manglano and Martin who studied the safety of triple lumen catheters in critically ill patients and found that catheters could be safely left in place for up to 10 days with minimal risk of bacteremia (1). Indeed, an interesting study by Eyer et al., strongly suggested that *no* routine guidelines for timing CVC changes be made (2). These researchers found that catheter-related sepsis was not affected by the duration of catheter placement. The chance of a patient developing catheter sepsis was found to be .3% to .5%/catheter/day, regardless of catheter exchange protocols. Apparently, the patient's underlying severity of illness correlated most strongly with the incidence of catheter-related sepsis. Should a catheter change be necessary, Eyer et al. recommended that a guidewire exchange be used unless the skin site was infected.

If the timing of central line catheter changes is no longer an important question, then we should put it to rest and address other questions. The studies discussed above did not use a consistent method of catheter care. A variety of gauze and occlusive dressings were used and changed every 48 to 72 hours. The types of dressings used were not correlated to findings of sepsis. Thus, what dressings should be used, and when should they be changed.? This is another one of those old repetitive questions echoing through hospitals everywhere.

There is another issue. Past research has shown that peripheral venous catheters should be changed every 72 hours or the incidence of infection increases. Perhaps the generic studies supporting frequent peripheral line changes need to be replicated, using current aseptic techniques of catheter insertion and care. This is especially important, in light of the fact that most catheter-related sepsis is related to contamination by the patient's own skin flora. For this reason, the study by Maki and Ringer (Abstract 7–2) is important to review, because it provides interesting comparative data on various skin antiseptic agents.

Answers to the nagging questions presented here must be found. What is required is an analytic evaluation of all the current research data available on the subject addressed here. Eventually, the method with the least complications and expense should be used—no question about it!—C. Kessler, RN, MN, CCRN, CS

References

1. Manglano R, Martin M: Safety of triple lumen catheters in the critically ill. *Am Surg* 57:370–372, 1991.
2. Eyer S, Brummitt C, Crossley K, et al: Catheter-related sepsis: Prospective, randomized study of three methods of long-term catheter maintenance. *Crit Care Med* 18:1073–1079, 1990.

Prospective Randomised Trial of Povidone-Iodine, Alcohol, and Chlorhexidine for Prevention of Infection Associated with Central Venous and Arterial Catheters

Maki DG, Ringer M, Alvarado CJ (Univ of Wisconsin, Madison)

Lancet 338:339–343, 1991 7–2

Problem.—Septicemia is the outstanding life-threatening complication in patients with vascular catheters. More than 90% of all septicemias re-

Catheter-Related Infections

Characteristic	Antiseptic group: 10% povidone-iodine (n=227)	70% alcohol (n=227)	2% chlorhexidine (n=214)
Central venous catheters			
No studied	77	32	67
Local infection (%)	15 (19·5)	5 (15·6)	4 (5·9)*
With bacteraemia (%)	5 (6·5)	2 (6·3)	1 (1·5)
Arterial catheters			
No studied	150	195	147
Local infection (%)	6 (4·0)	6 (3·1)	1 (0·7)
With bacteraemia (%)	1 (0·7)	1 (0·5)	0
Overall			
No studied	227	227	214
Local infection (%)	21 (9·3)	11 (7·1†)	5 (2·3)‡
With bacteraemia (%)	6 (2·6)	3 (2·3†)	1 (0·5)
No of infecting organisms (bacteraemia)			
Coagulase-negative staphylococci	13 (1)	9 (2)	3§
Staphylococcus aureus	1 (1)	1 (1)	..
Gram-negative bacilli	6¶ (3)	..	2 (1)
Enterococcus	1 (1)	..	..
Candida species	1 (1)	1	..

* Compared with povidine-iodine group, odds ratio = .26; compared with other 2 groups combined, odds ratio = .28.
† Rate adjusted to reflect distribution of central venous and arterial catheters similar to other 2 groups.
‡ Compared with povidine-iodine group, odds ratio = .23; compared with other 2 groups combined, odds ratio = .32.
§ Compared with other 2 groups combined, *P* = .03.
¶ Compared with other 2 groups combined, *P* = .02.
(Courtesy of Maki DG, Ringer M, Alvarado CJ: *Lancet* 338:339–343, 1991.)

lated to the presence of an intravascular device occur in those with a central venous or arterial catheter.

Study Methods.—Three antiseptics used to disinfect central venous and arterial catheter insertion sites were compared in a prospective study that included 668 catheter insertions. Patients were randomized to receive 10% povidone-iodine, 70% alcohol, or 2% aqueous chlorhexidine for disinfection of the catheter site and for care of the site on alternate days.

Findings.—The length of time the catheters were inserted was comparable in all groups. Insertion sites were colonized mainly by coagulase-negative staphylococci. No more than 5% of catheter hubs in any group were contaminated. Both local infection and bacteremia were least frequent when chlorhexidine was applied (table). Only one of 14 infusion-related bacteremias occurred in a chlorhexidine-treated patient.

Nursing Implications.—The use of 2% aqueous chlorhexidine to disinfect the skin before inserting an intravascular device and for postinsertional care of the site can substantially lower the risk of device-related infection.

Comments: Intravascular device-related septicemia ("line-sepsis") is a frequent and unwanted visitor to critical care units. This potentially life-threatening complication is thought by many to be inevitable in the severely compromised patient, whose external integrity is breached by numerous invasive procedures and whose internal immunologic armament is ineffectual. Such pessimism, although understandable, may not be totally warranted. The findings of the study presented in this article require that we reexamine our current practices of cutaneous disinfection.

The patient's own skin flora are typically the invading pathogens. Chemical antiseptics such as 70% alcohol and 10% povidone-iodine have long been used to thwart invasion by microorganisms at these catheter insertion sites. However, these venerated antiseptics apparently come up short in comparison to the potent germicide, chlorhexidine-gluconate. Not only is chlorhexidine-gluconate remarkably effective against catheter-related sepsis, it is less painfully noxious than other cutaneous disinfectants and is safe for newborns.

Prudence is required, however, before we dash out to rewrite our hospital standards on intravascular site care. Although these findings strongly suggest that chlorhexidine should be considered as a first-line antiseptic for prevention of infection with percutaneously inserted intravascular devices of all types, further corroborative studies are required. Additionally, single-use packets of the germicide have not yet been commercially produced, making the antiseptic less "user-friendly." Still, there is room for optimism. We may not win the war against line-sepsis, but we may be able to reduce the "casualties of war."—C. Kessler, RN, MN, CCRN, CS

Nutritional Support in HIV Infection: A Multilevel Analysis

Bradley-Springer L (New Mexico AIDS Education and Training Center, Albuquerque)

Image: J Nurs Scholarship 23:155–159, 1991 7–3

Purpose.—Human immunodeficiency virus is a chronic, prolonged infectious process. Health care providers must begin to apply their understanding of other chronic diseases to the care and treatment of HIV-infected patients. Nutrition is a major component in the treatment of chronic conditions. In HIV infection, malnutrition may be one of the first indicators that the disease is progressing. Nutritional support in HIV infection was reviewed using a multilevel perspective, ranging from personal psychology to institutional/societal controls.

Findings.—Human immunodeficiency virus infection causes immune dysfunction and protein-calorie malnutrition, which is the most common cause of acquired immune deficiency in humans. A vicious circle begins: HIV infection causes malnutrition, and malnutrition reduces immune function; opportunistic disease appears, adding to the stress on nutritional status. Causes of wasting in HIV-infected patients are related to intake interference, absorption problems, or a hypermetabolic state resulting from the infectious process. The range of nutritional problems associated with HIV infection and immune deficiency include increased levels of cachectin or tumor necrosis factor; hypertriglyceridemia independent of degree of wasting; depletion of potassium, body fat content, serum protein concentration and intracellular water volume; and progressive depletion of body cell mass. Also reported are reduced albumin and increased total serum protein levels, reduced iron binding capacity and selenium deficiency, and periods of hypometabolism in response to body cell mass depletion and nutrient malabsorption. Stressors that are caused by infection exacerbate these nutritional problems.

Conclusions.—Health care providers must consider the nutritional needs of HIV-infected patients. To provide holistic, economic, and supportive care to HIV-infected patients, nutritional assessment, diagnosis, and education must be integrated at the personal, interpersonal, organizational, and societal levels.

Comments: People who have HIV infection require holistic body-mind-spirit care. Because nurses spend more time with these patients than do any other health care professionals, they are in key positions to consider the multiple needs of patients. Adequate nutrition is essential for all physiologic functions, including the immune response. The immune system is compromised in HIV disease as a result of both the viral infection and inadequate nutrition. Opportunistic infections further compromise the immune system and nutritional status. Thus, HIV infection leads to compromised immune function, which leads to opportunistic infections which, in turn, further compromise the immune system. Finally, the appetite and food intake decrease, a wasting syndrome develops, and the immune system is further compromised. Although the immune status of the person with HIV disease cannot be returned to normal, its function may be supported with adequate nutrition. Food intake involves physiologic, social, spiritual, and other cultural parameters that can be assessed from personal, interpersonal, environmental, and societal levels. To enhance food intake and nutritional status of people with HIV disease, the nurse needs to assess the patient from each of these perspectives and then collaborate with the patient, physician, and nutritionist to plan an acceptable dietary regimen. Although the outcome of the assessing and planning may not increase the length of life for persons with HIV disease, it can improve the quality of their life. In a disease process that currently leads to a prolonged dying experience, any intervention that can improve the quality of that experience is worthwhile.—L.E. Lancaster, RN, MSN, EdD

Monitoring Universal Precautions: A New Assessment Tool

Gauthier DK, Turner JG, Langley LG, Neil CJ, Rush PL (Univ of Alabama, Birmingham)

Infect Control Hosp Epidemiol 12:597–601, 1991 7–4

Problem.—The Occupational Safety and Health Administration mandated that employers take specific steps to protect their employees from accidental exposures to blood-borne disease. Two important steps are the education of employees in the use of universal precautions (UP) and the provision of protective equipment needed to implement UPs. However, health care workers often fail to follow UP guidelines. An observational instrument was designed to determine a person's application of UPs in a clinical setting accurately and consistently.

Study Methods.—The instrument has a checklist format to elicit information on the use of barrier precautions, handwashing, proper disposal of needles and other sharp instruments, and the use of ventilation equipment to avoid mouth-to-mouth contact (Fig 7–1). In using the Universal Precautions Assessment Tool (UPAT), each opportunity for a health care worker to use UP whether the procedure is followed is noted by an observer. The UPAT was tested by 2 simultaneous observers to establish interrater reliability. The first pilot study was conducted in 3 different units within a 100-bed U.S. Army hospital and the second pilot study was conducted in the emergency department of a large university-based hospital.

Findings.—Two simultaneous raters determined UP compliance rates of 76.4% and 78.6%, respectively, for 9 nurses in the first pilot and 62% and 65% for 5 nurses in the second study.

Conclusion.—The UPAT was found to have an acceptable level of reliability. The advantages of the UPAT include avoiding the bias that might be present in self-reporting and providing a comprehensive UP compliance assessment. Limitations include the possibility of a Hawthorne effect and the fact that evaluating proper UP implementation sometimes relies on a "judgment call" by the observer. Testing conditions can be adjusted to minimize these effects to measure UP compliance.

Comments: Although the importance of universal precautions in preventing spread of blood-borne diseases is well recognized, it is difficult to monitor and assess health care workers' actual use of the precautions. The tool presented in this article provides such a method. The results of such a study could be used to update protocols and to point to the need for review of existing protocols. The results also could be used to provide feedback to nurses on those units that have high risks for blood-borne pathogen exposure. The feedback could either be presented to all of the nurses collectively or used for individual nurse guidance. The assessment tool was not designed specifically for nursing staff; therefore, it could be useful for other members of the

UNIVERSAL PRECAUTIONS ASSESSMENT TOOL

I. BARRIER PRECAUTIONS	GLOVE	MASK	EYES	GOWN
A. Blood (start IV, venipuncture, blood from art. line, fingerstick, etc.)				
B. Any body fluid with visible blood				
C. Other body fluids (no visible blood)				
Vaginal secretions				
Semen				
CSF				
Pleural, peritoneal, pericardial, synovial fluid				
Amniotic fluid				
Tissue specimen				
D. Mucous Membrane (eye, mouth, vag., rectal, NGtube insert, etc.)				
E. Surgery (Glove, mask req.)(major or minor)				
F. Non-intact skin (open wound, dress. change, etc.)				
G. OB (Glove, gown req.) (placenta, infant before washing, cord care)				

II. HANDWASHING

A. After contamination of skin

B. After removal of gloves

III. DISPOSAL OF SHARPS

A. Proper handling of used needles (not recapped or manipulated by hand)

B. Needles and other sharp instruments discarded in puncture-resistant container

Key: Y / N

IV. RESUSCITATION AND VENTILATION DEVICES used to avoid mouth to mouth contact

Unit: ________ Nurse code: ________ Score (Y / Y+N) x 100: ________

Time begin: ________ Time end: ________ Total time: ________ Date: ________

No. of patients cared for: ________ Observer: ________

Fig 7–1.—Universal Precautions Assessment Tool. (Courtesy of Gauthier DK, Turner JG, Langley LG, et al: *Infect Control Hosp Epidemiol* 12:597–601, 1991.)

health care team. One caution is that it must be made clear that the results of the study will not be used punitively, but rather to provide guidance, identify problems, and improve the use of universal precautions.—L.E. Lancaster, RN, MSN, EdD

Procedure-Related Rate of Contact of Intensive Care Unit Personnel With Patient Body Fluids

Kristensen, MS, Sloth E, Jensen TK (Randers Central Hospital, Denmark)
Intensive Care Med 17:276–280, 1991 7–5

Problem.—The universal precautions for health care workers to avoid HIV infection suggest focusing on procedures that involve risk of body fluid contact and considering all patients potentially infective. The procedure-related frequency of contact with blood and other body fluids among intensive care unit (ICU) personnel was studied to provide a basis for appropriate precautions.

Study Methods and Findings.—Personnel in the ICU filled out a questionnaire that contained 29 standardized procedures. Contact with body fluids of the patient occurred in 52% of instances when personnel were performing common ICU procedures. The most frequent fluids encountered were saliva and blood, followed by urine, tracheal secretions, stomach contents, feces, hemofiltrate, wound secretions, tears, and cerebrospinal fluid. The overall frequency of needlestick injuries was 0%.

Discussion.—Past research has shown that saliva contains HIV in 1% of HIV-seropositive patients. No seroconversions have been reported in persons bitten by AIDS patients. The Centers for Disease Control consider that the risk of HIV transmission through saliva is negligible unless it contains visible blood, but they also state that saliva should be considered infective for dental patients. Tracheal tubes and suction catheters used during general anesthesia often contain saliva and blood, which suggests that saliva and tracheal secretions encountered at this time should be considered potentially infective. Personnel must avoid all contact with blood. Cerebrospinal fluid contains HIV in 62.5% of seropositive patients, but infection through this fluid has not been reported. The Centers for Disease Control recommend using the same precautions in contacts with CSF of patients as is used in contacts with blood. Feces, tears, sweat, urine, and vomitus are also potentially infective if they contain visible blood.

Comments: Who comes in contact with more potentially HIV-infected body fluids than critical care nurses as they perform their day-to-day nursing care? Protective measures can be inadequate (health care workers have become infected) or over used, and they are very expensive and time consuming. Yet, the cost cannot be an issue if even 1 health care worker is saved from becoming HIV-infected by using appropriate precautions. The results of this study can be used to identify those procedures that are most likely to lead to contact with body fluids and the specific part of the caregiver's body that is most likely to contact the body fluid. Guidelines for those procedures, then can be developed to ensure adequate precautions. Thus, the use of gloves, long sleeves, masks, and protective eyewear can be determined for each procedure based on the potential for body fluid contact and the area of the body that is most susceptible to contact. Such a research-based approach can save money and time and can relieve the uncertainty of the health care worker about appropriate precautions for specific procedures.—L.E. Lancaster, RN, MSN, EdD

An Analysis of Blood and Body Fluid Exposures Sustained by House Officers, Medical Students, and Nursing Personnel on Acute-Care General Medical Wards: A Prospective Study

Stotka JL, Wong ES, Williams DS, Stuart CG, Markowitz SM (Med College of Virginia, Richmond; Hunter Holmes McGuire Dept of VA Med Ctr, Richmond, Va)

Infect Control Hosp Epidemiol 12:583–590, 1991 7–6

Problem.—Health care workers exposed to infected blood and body fluids are at risk for serious infections.

Study Methods.—The epidemiology of blood and body fluid exposures in medical house staff, medical students, registered nurses (RNs), licensed practical nurses (LPNs), and nurses' aides (NAs) on general medicine wards of 2 tertiary referral hospitals was studied prospectively with regard to problem areas that could be amenable to change.

TABLE 1.—Body Fluids Associated With Adverse Exposure for Nurses

Body Fluid	RN (%)	LPN (%)	Aide (%)	All Nurses (%)
Blood (non-needlestick)	118 (84.3)	13 (56.5)	29 (40.3)	160 (68.1)
Blood via needlestick	6 (4.3)	0 (0.0)	1 (1.4)	7 (3.0)
Wound drainage	1 (0.7)	5 (21.7)	25 (34.7)	31 (13.2)
Cerebrospinal fluid	0 (0.0)	0 (0.0)	0 (0.0)	0 (0.0)
Urine (hematuria)	3 (2.1)	1 (4.3)	8 (11.1)	12 (5.1)
Respiratory secretions	4 (2.9)	4 (17.4)	1 (1.4)	9 (3.8)
Pleural fluid	2 (1.4)	0 (0.0)	1 (1.4)	3 (1.3)
Peritoneal fluid	1 (0.7)	0 (0.0)	1 (1.4)	2 (0.9)
Other	5 (3.6)	0 (0.0)	6 (8.3)	11 (4.7)
Subtotal	140 (100)	23 (100)	72 (100)	
Total				235 (100)

* Difference among nursing status by logistic regression is $P = .0001$.

† All physician data (residents, interns, and medical students) are combined because the difference by status is not statistically different.

‡ Synovial fluid, melena, or not specified.

(Courtesy of Stotka JL, Wong ES, Williams DS, et al: *Infect Control Hosp Epidemiol* 12:583–590, 1991.)

TABLE 2.—Procedures Associated With Adverse Exposures for Nurses

	Nursing Status*			
Procedure	**RN (%)**	**LPN (%)**	**Aide (%)**	**All Nurses (%)**
IV insertion and care	93 (66.4)	7 (30.4)	17 (23.6)	117 (49.8)
Patient care†	13 (9.3)	9 (39.1)	46 (63.9)	68 (28.9)
Glucometer fingerstick	20 (14.3)	3 (13.0)	1 (1.4)	24 (10.2)
Other‡	14 (10.0)	4 (17.4)	8 (11.1)	26 (11.1)
Subtotal	140 (100)	23 (100)	72 (100)	
Total				**235 (100)**

* Difference among status by logistic regression is $P = .0001$.
† Wound care, cleaning patient or patient area.
‡ Foley catheter insertion, venipuncture, respiratory suctioning, arterial puncture, nasogastric tube manipulation, or assisting with thoracentesis or paracentesis.
(Courtesy of Stotka JL, Wong ES, Williams DS, et al: *Infect Control Hosp Epidemiol* 12:583–590, 1991.)

Findings.—Physicians reported 644 exposures, of which 98 (15.2%) were sustained by medicine residents, 296 (46%) by interns, and 250 (38.8%) by students. There was blood contact in 591 (91.8%) exposures. Among physicians, 575 (89.3%) exposures occurred during venipuncture, intravenous catheter manipulation, and arterial punctures. Interns and students were most often exposed during venipunctures and intravenous manipulations. Residents were most often exposed during emergency intravenous catheter placements. Of the exposures, 522 (81%) occurred between 7 AM and 7 PM. During 524 (81.4%) exposures, physicians were not using barrier devices. Nurses reported 235 exposures, of which 140 (59.6%) were sustained by RNs, 23 (9.8%) by LPNs, and 72 (30.6%) by NAs. The RNs' exposures frequently occurred during intravenous manipulations and glucometer fingersticks. A higher percentage of LPN and NA exposures occurred during nonprocedural patient care. Blood contact accounted for 167 (71.1%) and wound drainage accounted for 31 (13.2%) of exposures (Tables 1 and 2).

Nursing Implications.—Health care workers on general medicine wards are frequently exposed to blood and body fluids. Efforts to reduce exposures should be aimed at improving procedural skills of health care workers for venipunctures intravenous catheter insertions, and glucometer fingersticks, and at increasing the use of barrier devices during both procedural and nonprocedural tasks.

Comments: If you need research support for your policies and procedures related to infectious disease control, especially blood-borne pathogens, you will want to read this article and make it available to all the patient care staff on your unit. The results of the study certainly stress the importance of universal precautions in preventing the spread of blood-borne pathogens. The study results point to the number of accidental exposures because of poor procedural skills. This information supports the need for ongoing review of precautions related to procedures that are likely to expose health care workers to blood and other body fluids. The tables included in this abstract indicate the body fluids and procedures associated with adverse exposures for nurses. Thus, perhaps these are the procedures that require the most intense and frequent review of technique and safety.—L.E. Lancaster, RN, MSN, EdD

Management Guidelines for Health Care Workers Exposed to Blood and Body Fluids

Go GW, Baraff LJ, Schriger DL (UCLA School of Medicine, UCLA Med Ctr)

Ann Emerg Med 20:1341–1350, 1991 7–7

Problem.—Accidental exposure to potentially infectious blood and body fluids is an occupational hazard for health care workers. Specific management guidelines were reviewed for the immediate and subsequent treatment of health care personnel after such exposures. The guidelines are based on a collective review of the literature and recommendations of the Advisory Committee on Immunization Practices (ACIP). The guidelines cover only hepatitis B, hepatitis C, and HIV infection (Figs 7–2 and 7–3).

General Recommendations.—All health care workers should be instructed to seek immediate medical attention as soon as possible after parenteral exposure to blood and body fluids that are potentially infectious. The emergency department and occupational health department need to agree to follow the same set of management guidelines. Personnel with parenteral exposures should be referred to occupational health departments for follow-up when initial treatment was provided in the emergency department. Specific, detailed information must be obtained on the nature of the exposure, the source, and the person exposed. A checklist or complaint-specific medical record must be used to assure that all information is collected and recorded.

Comments: Despite the amount of stress on universal precautions and the care with which each health care worker tries to implement them, accidental exposure to blood and body fluids from infected patients will inevitably occur. Thus, guidelines for management of these accidental exposures are essential. Although the critical care nurse does not actually prescribe the treatment, he or she could serve on a multidisciplinary committee that collaborates on writing a protocol for such exposures. This article, while not proposing to provide the final word in treatment, does provide helpful guidelines and checklists for management of 3 blood-borne pathogens that currently cause much concern; that is, hepatitis B, hepatitis C, and HIV infection. Figures 7–2 and 7–3 included in the abstract provide a review of immediate emergency care and long-term occupational health follow-up treatment. The guidelines could be adopted as presented or modified for each hospital. As

1. Wound care/First aid
   A. Irrigate wound with normal saline or sterile water.
   B. Flush mucous membranes with water or saline.
   C. Injuries requiring suturing or other intervention should be treated as usual.
2. Tetanus prophylaxis
   A. Tetanus and diphtheria toxoids (Td): 0.5 mg IM if $\geq$ 10 years since last immunization.
   B. Tetanus immune globulin: Not required.
3. Laboratory evaluation
   A. Source patient (if known)
      1. HBsAg
      2. AntiHIV: The source's physician should be the one who requests and explains the reason for the HIV test and obtains consent.
   B. Exposed HCW
      1. AntiHBs
      2. AntiHIV (with HCW's consent)
4. Hepatitis B prophylaxis
   A. Source HBsAg positive or high risk (dialysis patient, IV drug user, etc):
      1. Exposed unvaccinated and not known antiHBs positive:
         a. Hepatitis B vaccine: 1.0 mL IM. Second and third immunizations in one and six months at occupational health as function of serologic results on exposed.
         b. HBIG: 0.06 mL/kg IM.
      2. Exposed vaccinated and known responder (antiHBs $\geq$ 10 mIU) or immune status unknown
         a. No HBV vaccine or HBIG in ED. Treatment at occupational health as dictated by serologic results on source and exposed.
      3. Exposed vaccinated and known responder (antiHBs $\leq$ 10 mIU):
         a. Hepatitis B vaccine: 1.0 mL IM.
         b. HBIG: 0.06 mL/kg IM.
   B. Source HBsAg negative, low-risk or unknown
      1. Exposed unvaccinated and not known antiHBs positive:
         a. Hepatitis B vaccine: 1.0 mL IM. Second and third immunizations in at one and six months at occupational health as function of serologic results on exposed.
         b. HBIG: Not indicated. Treatment at occupational health as function of serologic results on source and exposed.
      2. Exposed vaccinated
         No hepatitis B vaccine or HBIG in ED. Treatment at occupational health as function of serologic results on source and exposed.
5. Hepatitis C prophylaxis
   If source antiHCV positive or HBsAg negative chronic hepatitis:
      Immune globulin: If exposed not to receive HBIG, then IG (0.06 mL/kg IM).
6. HIV prophylaxis
   A. General information:
      Zidovudine, if indicated (see below) should be prescribed only after discussion of risks, benefits, and alternatives. All patients should receive and read the *HCW Information: Occupational Exposure to Blood and Body Fluids.* All patients with parenteral exposures to blood or body fluid from a known HIV-positive source, or a source that is likely to be HIV positive, should be given the opportunity to take zidovudine. If the source patient is judged to be at high risk for HIV infection and the HIV antibody status is unknown or pending, the exposed should be treated until the results of this test are known. It is better to start therapy for HCWs who are unsure what to do, and discontinue it 48 to 72 hours later than to delay therapy. If the exposure warrants therapy, give zidovudine 200 mg as soon as possible. Then prescribe a three-day supply:

Rx Zidovudine 100-mg tabs #36 Sig: Tab 2 Q4H

   B. Zidovudine eligibility criteria
      1. Inclusion criteria
         a. Source of exposure
            1. Blood and all bloody body fluids from individuals with clinically diagnosed AIDS or AIDS-related complex, who are HIV antibody positive or are in a high-risk group (pending HIV testing).
            2. Fluids or tissues contaminated with high concentrations of HIV in research laboratories that have not been physically or chemically inactivated.
         b. Type of exposure
            1. Substantial exposure (zidovudine encouraged)
               a. Injections of contaminated blood.
               b. Parenteral exposure to laboratory materials containing high titers of HIV.
            2. Definite exposure (zidovudine offered)
               a. Laceration or needlestick produced by a contaminated sharp instrument that causes bleeding.
               b. Laceration or similar fresh wound inoculated with contaminated blood or bloody body fluid.
            3. Low-risk exposure (zidovudine not routinely recommended)
               a. Superficial (nonbleeding) injury with contaminated needle or instrument.
               b. Mucous membrane exposure.
               c. Time of exposure: Treatment should begin within 48 hours of exposure to HIV-infected material.
      2. Exclusion criteria
         a. Prior diagnosis of HIV infection in exposed.
         b. Underlying renal insufficiency (creatinine > 3.0).
         c. Underlying hepatic insufficiency (ALT, alkaline phosphatase, or total bilirubin > 5 times normal).
         d. Bone marrow dysfunction (Hgb < 9 g/dL); granulocytes < 1,000/mm^3).
         e. Pregnancy
   C. Additional laboratory evaluation for HCWs given zidovudine
      Pregnancy test
      CBC, differential, platelet count
      Creatinine
      ALT, alkaline phosphatase, total bilirubin
7. Follow-up evaluation
   A. Occupational health: All patients should be instructed to report to occupational health in 48 to 72 hours. The following therapy will be provided.
      1. Counseling regarding the results of the serologic studies drawn from the HCW and the source.
      2. Completion of hepatitis B immunization when indicated.
      3. HBIG (if not already administered) when the source is found to be HBsAg positive and the exposed is antiHBs negative.
      4. Decision whether to continue zidovudine therapy.

Fig 7–2.—Emergency department (immediate) treatment of needlestick and other exposures to blood and body fluids. (Courtesy of Go GW, Baraff LF, Schriger DL: *Ann Emerg Med* 20:1341–1350, 1991.)

1. Hepatitis B prophylaxis
   A. Source HBsAg positive and exposed antiHBs positive (antiHBs ≥ 10 mIU).
      1. No treatment necessary.
   B. Source HBsAg positive and exposed antiHBs negative (antiHBs < 10 mIU).
      1. Exposed vaccinated
         a. Hepatitis B vaccine: 1.0 mL IM if not given in ED.
         b. HBIG: 0.06 mL/kg IM if not given in ED.
      2. Exposed unvaccinated
         a. Hepatitis B vaccine: 1.0 mL IM if not given in ED. Second and third immunizations in one and six months.
         b. HBIG: 0.06 mL/kg IM if not given in ED.
   C. Source HBsAg negative and exposed antiHBs positive
      1. No treatment necessary.
   D. Source HBsAg negative and exposed antiHBs negative
      1. Exposed vaccinated
         a. Hepatitis B vaccine: 1.0 mL IM if not given in ED.
         b. AntiHBs in one month
            (1) If < 10 mIU: Exposed is partial or nonresponder
            (2) If ≥ 10 mIU: Exposed is immune
      2. Exposed unvaccinated
         a. Hepatitis B vaccine: 1.0 mL IM if not given in ED. Second and third immunizations in one and six months.
2. HIV prophylaxis
   A. General information: See Figure 2
   B. Zidovudine prophylaxis: Zidovudine is assumed to only be of value if begun within 48 hours of exposure. Therefore, it may be begun as part of the ED (initial) management of the (needlestick) exposure before the results of laboratory tests are known, and the decision to continue therapy is based on these results. If it has not been begun within 48 hours of exposure, it is probably too late to be of value.
      1. Source HIV positive and exposed HIV negative
         a. Continue AZT for four weeks. Prescribe additional medication:

            Rx

            Zidovudine 100-mg tabs
            #250
            Sig: Tab 2 Q4H, 5X/Day

         b. Refer for infectious disease consultation: Patients treated with zidovudine should be instructed to make an appointment with an infectious disease consultant involved in postexposure zidovudine treatment of HCWs. Each zidovudine-treated HCW must be evaluated by a clinician at two and four weeks when tests for zidovudine toxicity will be conducted. Repeat blood tests for HIV antibody should be done at four weeks, and three, six, and 12 months after exposure.
         c. If the source was not previously known to be HIV positive, be certain that the treating physician is aware of the test results.
      2. Source HIV negative and exposed HIV negative
         a. Discontinue zidovudine.
      3. Exposed HIV positive
         a. Inform HCW of results and provide counseling.
         b. Discontinue zidovudine.
         c. Refer to an infectious disease consultant with experience in treating AIDS for counseling and possible treatment.

Fig 7–3.—Occupational health (follow-up) treatment of needlestick and other exposures to blood and body fluids. (Courtesy of Go GW, Baraff LF, Schriger DL: *Ann Emerg Med* 20:1341–1350, 1991.)

for all protocols, the guidelines must be individualized based on specific patient assessment. In addition, ongoing revision of the guidelines is essential as new information and improved treatment options are available.—LE Lancaster, RN, MSN, EdD

8 Renal Dysfunction

Catheter-Associated Urinary Tract Infections: Epidemiology, Pathogenesis, and Prevention

Stamm WE (Harborview Med Ctr, Seattle)

Am J Med 913B÷65S–71S, 1991 8–1

Problem.—The most common nosocomial infection is catheter-associated urinary tract infection (UTI_c). These infections account for about 40% of infections in most hospitals.

Epidemiology.—The major risk factors for UTI_c are female gender, duration of catheterization, absence of systemic antibiotics, and catheter care violations. The case fatality rate for those with UTI_c is almost 3 times that for nonbacteriuric patients, probably because of secondary bacteremia and septicemia. Sealed junction catheters have been found to decrease significantly the risk of UTI in catheterized patients and the risk of death in patients not receiving systemic antimicrobials.

Pathogenesis.—Bacteria take the periurethral or intraluminal route of entry into the catheterized urinary tract. About 70% of episodes of bacteriuria in women occur through the periurethral route. Bacteria that infect the urinary tract in women usually emanate from rectal flora. In men most infections occur by the intraluminal route. Bacteria entering the urinary drainage bag can be found 24 to 48 hours later in the bladder, a phenomenon occurring with great regularity in patients not receiving antimicrobials. There are 2 populations of bacteria in the catheterized urinary tract, those growing within the urine itself and those growing on the surface of the catheter.

Prevention.—Staff education and behavior modification may play a role in reducing the occurrence of bacteriuria in hospitalized patients. The use of sealed junctions is an alternative approach. Systemic antimicrobials can reduce the occurrence of UTI_c in the first 4–5 days of catheterization. Systemic antimicrobials may be considered as a preventive measure in high-risk patients with an anticipated short duration of catheterization. A recent study has demonstrated the value of selective decontamination of the gut in preventing UTI_c.

Long-Term Catheterization.—The prevalence of bacteriuria in patients with long-term catheterization is essentially 100%. Intermittent urethral catheterization has been found to be effective, compared with long-term in-dwelling catheterization. It has not been possible to show the efficacy of any prophylactic regimen in patients with chronically indwelling catheters.

Conclusions.—Although UTI_c is usually benign, it can be fatal. Future research to help control the incidence of UTI_c most likely will focus on design of the urinary catheter system, bacterial-host epithelial cell interaction, and targeted antimicrobial prophylaxis.

Comments: It is almost expected that every critically ill patient routinely will have an indwelling urinary catheter. Although most hospitals have a routine catheter care protocol, catheter-associated urinary tract infections remain the most common nosocomial infection. The critically ill patient, who probably has a compromised immune response and is exposed to numerous pathogens, is particularly susceptible to such infections. As with all cases of infection, prevention is the best treatment.

Perhaps it is time for nurses, in collaboration with physicians, to evaluate the catheter care protocol based on current information about epidemiology, pathogenesis, and prevention of acute and long-term catheter-related infections. This article provides a very helpful overview of these areas and makes specific suggestions for preventing this prevalent problem. Thus, the article would serve as an invaluable guide for revising catheter care protocols. In addition, the section entitled Future Directions suggests many questions that could stimulate nursing and medical research about this major problem.—L.E. Lancaster, RN, MSN, EdD

Drug-Induced Renal Toxicity: Help in Recognizing Offending Agents

Farrugia E, Larson TS (Mayo Clinic and Found, Rochester, Minn)

Postgrad Med 90:241–248, 1991 8–2

Problem.—Renal toxicity is increasingly recognized as a complication of both diagnostic and therapeutic agents. A number of drug-induced nephrotoxic syndromes and their possible causes are shown in the table.

NSAIDs.—Acute renal failure induced by nonsteroidal anti-inflammatory drugs (NSAIDs) often is hemodynamically mediated, occurring when renal blood flow and glomerular filtration are dependent on the synthesis of renal vasodilatory prostaglandins. Renal insufficiency typically develops rapidly and is characterized by oliguria, progressive azotemia, and salt retention. Patients generally recover completely when the offending drug is withdrawn. These drugs must be avoided in patients at high risk or must be used for a short time in the lowest feasible dose.

Aminoglycosides.—These drugs can accumulate in the proximal renal tubule cells and damage them. Acute renal failure is less frequent and usually occurs in critically ill patients. Typically, acute nonoliguric renal failure develops within a week after initiation of therapy. Recovery may be slow or incomplete. The kidneys are the chief route for aminoglycoside elimination, and dosage must be adjusted according to the glomerular filtration rate.

Drug-Induced Nephrotoxic Syndromes

Disorder	Implicated Agents
Acute renal failure	
Prerenal azotemia	NSAIDs, ACE inhibitors, cyclosporine (Sandimmune), radiocontrast material, interleukin-2
Acute tubular cell necrosis	Aminoglycosides, heavy metals, amphotericin B (Fungizone) radiocontrast material, cisplatin (Platinol)
Intratubular obstruction	Acyclovir (Zovirax), radiocontrast material, methotrexate, sulfonamides
Acute myoglobinuric renal failure	Lovastatin (Mevacor), gemfibrozil (Lopid), heroin
Glomerulopathy	
Lipoid nephrosis	NSAIDs, alpha interferon
Membranous nephropathy	Gold, penicillamine (Cuprimine, Depen), captopril (Capoten)
Focal segmental glomerulosclerosis	Heroin
Obstructive uropathy	
Urolithiasis	Acetazolamide (Diamox), allopurinol (Lopurin, Zyloprim), triamterene (Dyrenium)
Retroperitoneal fibrosis	Methysergide maleate (Sansert)
Vascular or microvascular disease	
Hemolytic-uremic syndrome	Mitomycin (Mutamycin), cyclosporine
Vasculitis	Allopurinol, sulfonamides
Tubulointerstitial nephritis	
Acute interstitial nephritis	Beta-lactam antibiotics, NSAIDs, sulfonamides, allopurinol, cimetidine (Tagamet), rifampin (Rifadin, Rimactane), diuretics
Chronic renal failure (chronic tubulointerstitial nephropathy)	Aspirin and acetaminophen (ie, analgesic nephropathy), cyclosporine, heavy metals, lithium
Fluid and electrolyte disorders	
Renal tubular acidosis	Amphotericin B, acetazolamide, outdated tetracycline HCI
Nephrogenic diabetes insipidus	Lithium
Hyperkalemia	ACE inhibitors, cyclosporine, NSAIDs
Hyponatremia	NSAIDs, thiazide diuretics
Hypomagnesemia	Aminoglycosides, cisplatin, amphotericin B
Hypocalcemia	Cisplatin
Hypokalemia	Thiazide diuretics, aminoglycosides

(Courtesy of Farrugia E, Larson TS: *Postgrad Med* 90:241–248, 1991.)

Angiotensin-Converting Enzyme (ACE) Inhibitors.—These drugs are able to induce acute, reversible renal dysfunction in patients with renovascular stenosis. Vasoregulation may be compromised by a single dose of an ACE inhibitor. The drugs must be used cautiously in those who are at risk for renovascular disease. If azotemia develops during treatment, the drug must be withdrawn.

Radiocontrast Materials.—Intravascular contrast injections may cause up to 12% of cases of acute renal failure in hospitalized patients. Diabetic patients with renal insufficiency are especially at risk. Oliguric renal failure often develops immediately after contrast administration. If possible, an alternative procedure such as ultrasonography or MRI is used in patients at high risk. The chief means of preventing radiocontrast-induced renal failure is adequate hydration.

Comments: I think most nurses and health professionals in general are unaware that almost any drug can be nephrotoxic if the drug is given in high dosages or if the patient has preexisting compromised kidney function. Most critically ill patients, especially the very young, the elderly, and those with multisystem problems, are likely to have compromised kidney function and, therefore, can develop drug-induced renal toxicity more rapidly and in reponse to lower drug dosages than healthy individuals. Thus, it is the critical care nurses' responsibility to assess each patient's kidney function status (BUN, serum creatinine, creatinine clearance, urine output) and the potential nephrotoxic effects of all drugs the patient is receiving. This article provides an excellent overview of 4 groups of potential nephrotoxic substances that are often used to treat inflammation, infection, hypertension, and congestive heart failure. The article is particularly helpful because it discusses each group of potentially nephrotoxic substances in terms of risk factors that can potentiate renal toxicity and clinical features of nephrotoxicity. Prevention of drug-induced kidney damage, which is the most important approach to the problem, is thoroughly summarized. The article will assist critical care nurses in the assessment and recognition of potential or actual drug-induced renal toxicity and collaboration with physicians and pharmacists for prevention and early management.—L.E. Lancaster, RN, MSN, EdD

9 Transplantation and Immunology

The Present and Future of Kidney Transplantation
Najarian JS, Matas AJ (Univ of Minnesota, Minneapolis)
Transplant Proc 23:2075–2082, 1991 9–1

Purpose.—In the United States, approximately 9,000 patients undergo kidney transplant operations each year. Post-operative care for kidney transplant patients and the potential posttransplant complications were reviewed.

Postoperative Care.—Kidney transplant recipients always require intensive care support in the immediate posttransplant period. Although most patients are extubated at the completion of the operation, all require 1-to-1 nursing care for the first 24 hours. Vital signs must be monitored every 15 minutes until stable and then hourly thereafter. When a pulmonary artery catheter is placed, central venous and pulmonary artery pressures are measured hourly. Fluid and electrolyte status must be monitored. Urine output is measured and replaced milliliter for milliliter for the first 24 hours. Electrolytes are replaced as needed. Fluid replacement in patients with massive diuresis represents a large glucose load, and levels of blood sugar in both diabetic and nondiabetic patients need to be monitored. Hyperglycemia can be corrected by switching from a dextrose plus saline intravenous fluid replacement solution to a saline solution. Levels of phosphorus and magnesium must be checked daily. After the first 24 hours, volume replacement is gradually tapered until maintenance replacement levels are reached.

Postoperative Medications.—All patients are treated with immunosuppressive drugs, which may include prednisone, cyclosporine A, azathioprine, and antilymphocyte globulin. However, treatment protocols vary by institution. For the first 3 postoperative days patients are often treated with antibiotics to reduce the incidence of urinary tract infections, acyclovir to prevent cytomegalovirus infection, nystatin to prevent *Candida* infection, and a diuretic to counteract sodium retention associated with prednisone. Antacids to reduce stomach acidity are given every 2–4 hours.

Complications.—Potential complications are atelectasis, line sepsis, wound complications, pneumonia, bleeding, and oligoanuria. Although the incidence of these complications is relatively low, any complication is a cause for concern because of the patient's immunosuppressed status.

Arterial thrombosis is rare, but it usually results in graft loss. A high level of creatinine is probably the most common complication, and it may be the first indication that the transplant is being rejected. It also may represent other problems, including nephrotoxicity from cyclosporine A or other drugs, infection, recurrent disease, arterial stenosis, hyperglycemia, ureteral obstruction, or lymphocele. Immunosuppressive agents are associated with individual complications. An increased risk of infection, particularly opportunistic infection, remains a major problem with all immunosuppressive agents.

Comments: Kidney transplants have been performed longer and more successfully than any other solid organ or tissue transplant. Yet, thorough preoperative preparation and intensive postoperative management of these patients are essential to enhance success of the transplant and to prevent complications. Nurses are involved throughout all phases of kidney transplantation—from preoperative evaluation to the intensive care phase to long-term follow-up. Although this article does not provide an in-depth discussion of the medical or nursing intervention for any one particular phase, it does provide an excellent overview of the entire spectrum of kidney transplantation. The sections on the postoperative intensive care phase, postoperative medication and immunosuppression regimens, and postoperative technical and immunosuppression complications are particularly suited to the needs of critical care nurses. Because there are many reasons for an elevated serum creatinine level after transplant, the guidelines for assessing reasons for its elevation are helpful. Because many kidney transplant patients are debilitated from the prolonged period of end-stage renal disease, they are particularly susceptible to postoperative complications related to the transplant surgery and complications secondary to the immunosuppression regimen. Critical care nurses are the ones who assess the immediate posttransplant patient most often and therefore they need to understand the common complications and related assessment findings. These are comprehensively summarized in the article.

This article is important reading for all critical care nurses who care for transplant recipients and for nurses who care for patients during their long-term management.—L.E. Lancaster, RN, MSN, EdD

The Impact of Infection on the Outcome of Transplantation

Rubin RH, Tolkoff-Rubin NE (Massachusetts Gen Hosp, Boston; Harvard Univ, Boston)

Transplant Proc 23:2068–2074, 1991 9–2

Purpose.—The risk of infection in an organ transplant recipient is determined by the patient's net state of immunosuppression and by the environmental exposures the patient encounters. Interaction between these 2 determinants may cause a series of clinical syndromes that are unique to transplant patients. The clinical and epidemiologic characteristics of these syndromes were reviewed.

Immunosuppressive Therapy.—A review of the published literature suggested the following guidelines: When the effects of an immunosuppressive program on the occurrence of posttransplant infection are being assessed, all components of that program must be evaluated. When 1 very potent antirejection drug is used, the dosage of the other agents in the program needs to be decreased. By analyzing how an immunosuppressive program promotes particular infections, antibiotics that prevent those infections can be administered simultaneously as part of the immunosuppressive program.

Infection Timetable.—Three distinct posttransplant time periods, each with different infectious disease problems, have been identified. During the first month after transplant, infections that were present before transplant may be exacerbated by the posttransplant immunosuppression. For 1–6 months after transplant, infection with cytomegalovirus (CMV), Epstein-Barr virus, hepatitis viruses, and HIV may occur. Viral infection also may enable superinfection with opportunistic organisms such as *Pneumocystis carinii*, *Listeria monocytogenes*, and *Aspergillus* species. By 6 months or more after transplant, viral infections may have become chronic.

Viral Infections.—Viruses are of particular importance to the organ transplant patient. Cytomegalovirus has been linked with acute rejection and chronic coronary atherosclerosis in heart transplant patients, obliterative bronchiolitis in lung transplant patients, acute liver injury and chronic disappearing bile duct syndrome in liver transplant patients, and glomerulopathy in renal transplant patients. Hepatitis C infection is almost always chronic and almost always leads to end-stage liver disease. Transmission of HIV by transplantation of an infected organ is a growing, although totally preventable, problem for transplant patients.

Other Infections.—Transplant recipients also are pront to the development of bacterial and fungal infections (e.g., pneumonia caused by infection with the fungus *P. carinii* occurs in 5% of all transplant patients).

Current Status.—Because prevention of infection in transplant recipients is far better than treatment, antimicrobial prophylaxis and preemptive therapy are being increasingly used to blunt the unique complications of intensive antirejection therapy.

Comments: Organ and tissue transplant patients are caught in a double bind. Without immunosuppressive medications, they can reject their organ transplant, and with them they are subject to numerous complications, particularly infection. Prevention or early recognition and treatment of posttransplant infections can mean the difference between life and death for these patients.

Opportunistic infections that occur primarily in immunosuppressed patients are especially prevalent in the posttransplant period. Because immunosuppressed posttransplant patients require a lengthy stay in the critical care unit and on a general surgical unit, they are susceptible to nosocomial infections. Critical care nurses work as part of a collaborative organ transplant team in the prevention, recognition, administration of organism-specific medications, and assessment of desired and adverse effects of treatment. Thus, they must be knowledgeable about typical infective organisms related to specific immunosuppressive agents and protocols, signs and symptoms specific to each type of infection, pharmacology of medications, and long-term assessment of the effects of the infection and its treatment. In addition, the effects of the infections and their treatment on the outcome of the organ transplant must be considered.

This article provides comprehensive guidelines to nurses and other members of the organ transplant team. It could be used as a basis for developing a standardized protocol for assessing and treating infection related to organ transplantation. It could also be used as the basis for an infection surveillance program for any group of patients who require immunosuppression.—L.E. Lancaster, RN, MSN, EdD

Orthoclone OKT3: An Overview of the Monoclonal Antibody and the Nursing Considerations It Presents

Pezze JL, Whiteman K (Presbyterian Univ Hosp, Pittsburgh)

Crit Care Nurse 11:98–107, 1991 9–3

Mechanisms of Action.—Orthoclone OKT3 (muromonab CD3), the first monoclonal antibody to be used widely in clinical transplantation, is a murine antibody specific to the CD3 antigen on the surface of human T cells. This antibody alters the cell-mediated immune response by blocking the activation and function of mature T cells through an action on CD3, which is located next to the antigen recognition complex on T cells. Circulating CD3-bearing T cells rapidly disappear from the circulation within minutes of the initial OKT3 injection; the cells later reappear without the CD3 molecule and antigen recognition complex.

Clinical Uses.—Orthoclone OKT3 can reverse acute rejection of renal, cardiac, hepatic, and pancreatic transplants. Both primary treatment and rescue therapy are effective. The use of OKT3 in place of cyclosporine lowers the risks of hypertension, CNS toxicity, and nephrotoxicity. Additionally, OKT3 has proved helpful in treating acute graft-vs.-host disease after bone marrow transplantation.

Adverse Effects.—Most sequelae (table) occur within an hour of the initial dose of OKT3 when CD3-bearing T cells are most abundant. Lysis of these cells releases vasoactive mediators that produce systemic inflammation and constitutional symptoms such as fever, nausea-vomiting, and diarrhea. Pulmonary edema and aseptic meningitis are comparatively infrequent effects. Infections are most frequent within 45 days of the start of treatment.

Summary of OKT3

Action	Blocks the activation and function of mature T-cells
Indication	Primary prevention or treatment for acute transplant rejection
Contraindications	-Hypersensitivity to products of murine origin -Fluid overload -Anti-OKT3 antibody level greater than 1:100
Adverse Effects/ Reactions	-Reactions, such as fever, pulmonary edema, and anaphylaxis, usually occur 45-60 minutes after initial dose and can persist for several hours or more -These reactions occur to a lesser extent after the second dose -Effects, such as infections and aseptic meningitis, may occur later (during or after therapy)
Mild	Fever, chills, dyspnea, chest pain, vomiting, wheezing, nausea, diarrhea, tremor, weakness, anorexia, headaches, hyper/hypotension, pruritus, rash, nightmares, nasal and ear stuffiness, rigors
Severe or Rare	Anaphylaxis, pulmonary edema, infection (CMV, herpes simplex, staphylococcus epidermidis, pneumocystis carinii, legionella, cyptococcus, serratia, and gram negative bacteria), aseptic meningitis, hearing loss, serum sickness, lymphoma, Epstein-Barr virus, seizures, monarticular arthritis, transient ischemic attacks, acute renal artery thrombosis, subarachnoid hemorrhage, acute psychosis, Guillain-Barre-like syndrome
Dosage	5 mg (5 cc) per day for 10-14 days
Nursing Implications	-Premedicate as prescribed -Epinephrine 1:10,000 and diphenhydramine hydrochloride available in case of anaphylaxis -Monitor vital signs before and after administration -See example in Table 5

Abbreviation: CMV, cytomegalovirus.
(Courtesy of Pezze JL, Whiteman K, *Crit Care Nurse* 11:98–107, 1991.)

Nursing Implications.—Orthoclone OKT3 is given by rapid (less than 1 minute) intravenous bolus injection, not infusion. It is not administered with other drugs. The usual premedications include analgesia, an antipyretic, an antihistamine, and a steroid. The presence of fluid overload raises the risk of pulmonary edema after OKT3 injection.

Comments: The frequency of the various types of organ transplants is increasing yearly. For an organ transplant to be successful, immunosuppressive therapy is essential to block the recipient's immune system from rejecting the transplanted organ. During the early posttransplant period, the critical care nurse administers various immunosuppressive agents and monitors their desired effects and side effects. During the early posttransplant period, OKT3 has become one of the most frequently administered immunosuppressive agents. This comprehensive, yet thorough, article provides information that can be applied in many different nursing situations related to OKT3 administration. Because the article includes specific information about patient preparation, drug administration techniques, and patient assessment, it could be used as the basis for developing a standardized protocol or nursing care plan for both first-dose administration and long-term care. It would be an excellent tool for teaching new nurses and students about the manufacture and pharmacology of OKT3 and related nursing implications. The discussion and clear illustrations about the effects of OKT3 on specific aspects of the immune system aid in understanding its desired and adverse effects. The article is recommended reading for practicing critical care nurses, transplant nurses, nursing students, and teachers of students and practicing nurses.—L.E. Lancaster, RN, MSN, EdD

Management of Drug Interactions With Cyclosporine

Lake KD (Abbott Northwestern Hosp, Minneapolis)

Pharmacotherapy 11:110S-118S, 1991 9–4

Problem.—The use of cyclosporine (CsA) has allowed many of the major advances in transplantation and treatment of autoimmune disorders of recent years. However, throughout a decade of use, many agents have been reported to interact with CsA. The various types of interactions and their management are reviewed.

Interactions.—Interactions may be either pharmacokinetic or pharmacodynamic in nature. The pharmacokinetic types cause an increase or decrease in CsA concentration, usually through alterations in the cytochrome P-450 metabolism of CsA. Other drugs may affect the absorption, distribution, and elimination of CsA. In pharmacodynamic interactions, the pharmacologic or toxicologic effects of CsA are altered. These types of interactions include enhancement of nephrotoxicity. Other interactions may result in myalgia, myopathy, and rhabdomyolysis; gingival hyperplasia; or an altered immunologic effect (table).

Management.—When a CsA interaction is confirmed, proactive measures are needed. The interactive potential of each new agent must be assessed, CsA concentrations must be measured more often when new agents are introduced or discontinued, and dosage must be adjusted as necessary. Patients are monitored to ensure the efficacy and minimize the risk of CsA toxicity.

Conclusions.—The drug interactions seen with CsA and their management are presented. The clinical implications of these interactions may range from minor disturbances to graft rejection and nephrotoxicity. Generally, the pharmacodynamic interactions are harder to assess and predict.

Cyclosporin (CsA) Drug Interactions

Drug	Proposed Mechanism	Possible Effects	References
Anticonvulsants			
* Carbamazepine	Increased CsA metabolism	Decreased CsA blood concentrations	74, 75
Mesuximide	As above	As above	1
* Phenobarbital	As above	As above	72, 73
* Phenytoin	As above	As above	22, 23, 47
	Decreased CsA absorption	As above	19
Primidone	Increased CsA metabolism	As above	73, 76
Valproic acid	——	No effect	75
Antiinfective agents			
Acyclovir	Nephrotoxic agent	Increased nephrotoxicity	132
* Aminoglycosides	As above	Increased nephrotoxicity	129, 130
* Amphotericin B	As above	Increased nephrotoxicity	131
Cephalosporins	——	No effect (animal studies)	151
Ciprofloxacin	——	No effect	110–112
* Doxycycline	Unknown	Increased CsA concentrations	1
* Erythromycin	Decreased CsA metabolism	Increased CsA blood concentrations with and without nephrotoxicity	42–48
	Decreased biliary excretion	As above	48
	Increased absorption	As above	14–16
Fluconazole	Decreased CsA metabolism	Increased CsA concentrations (conflicting data)	101–103
Ganciclovir	Unknown	Increased nephrotoxicity	133
Imipenem-cilastatin	Increased CsA metabolism	Decreased CsA blood concentrations (animal studies)	114
	Unknown	Increased CsA concentrations with neurotoxicity	115
Itraconazole	Decreased CsA metabolism	Increased CsA blood concentrations (conflicting data)	97–100
* Josamycin	Decreased CsA metabolism	Increased CsA blood concentrations	93
* Ketoconazole	Decreased CsA metabolism	Increased CsA blood concentrations with and without nephrotoxicity	31, 34–41
* Nafcillin	Increased CsA metabolism	Decreased CsA blood concentration	88
Norfloxacin	Decreased CsA metabolism	Increased CsA concentrations (conflicting data)	113
Pristinamycin	Decreased CsA metabolism	Increased CsA concentration	1
Spiramycin	——	No effect	94–96
* Sulfamethoxazole and/or Trimethoprim			
* i.v.	Unknown	Decreased CsA blood concentrations with associated rejection episodes	86, 87
p.o.	Altered tubular secretion of creatinine	Increased serum creatinine	137
Ticarcillin	Unknown	Increased CsA concentrations	1
Antituberculous agents			
Isoniazid	Increased CsA metabolism(?)	Decreased CsA blood concentrations with with concomitant rifampin therapy	79
* Rifampin	As above	As above	76–85
Cardiovascular agents			
* Diltiazem	Decreased CsA metabolism	Increased CsA blood concentrations	50–59, 70
Disopyramide	Unknown	Increased serum creatinine	138
Enalapril	Unknown	Protective renal effect	146
* Nicardipine	Decreased CsA metabolism	Increased CsA blood concentrations	60–62
Nifedipine	——	No effect on CsA	56, 60, 66–68
	Unknown	Increased gingival hyperplasia	155–156

(continued)

Table *(continued)*

Drug	Proposed Mechanism	Possible Effects	References
Cardiovascular Agents (cont.)			
Nitrendipine	——	No effect on CsA	69
Prazosin	Improved renal blood flow	Protective renal effect (animal studies)	147
Propranolol	Unknown	Antagonistic immunosuppressive effect (animal studies)	123
* Verapamil	Decreased metabolism	Increased CsA concentrations	59, 63–65
	Unknown	Protective renal effect (animal studies)	148, 149
	Inhibits lymphocyte activation	Enhanced immunosuppression	157–159
Warfarin	Altered CsA metabolism in combination with phenobarbital	Decreased CsA concentrations and increased prothrombin activity	165
Diuretics			
Acetazolamide	Increased absorption Decreased metabolism Altered distribution	Increased CsA concentrations	32
Furosemide	Sodium depletion	Increased nephrotoxicity (animal studies)	143
		Protective renal effect	142
Mannitol	Unknown	Increased nephrotoxicity (animal studies)	145
Metolazone	Unknown	Increased nephrotoxicity	144
Spironolactone	Unknown	Protective renal effect (animal studies)	146
Gastrointestinal Agents			
Antacids	Decreased or increased absorption	Unknown,? similar to food (conflicting data)	9, 10, 22
Cholestyramine	Altered CsA absorption	Variable CsA concentrations or no effect	166
Cimetidine	Decreased CsA metabolism(?)	Increased CsA blood concentrations and/or nephrotoxicity (conflicting data)	123, 124, 126
	Altered tubular secretion of creatinine	Elevated serum creatinine	141
Famotidine	——	No effect	128
Lovastatin	Decreased lovastatin metabolism	Myositis, increased CPK, rhabdomyolysis	152–154
Metoclopramide	Increased CsA absorption	Increased CsA blood concentrations with nephrotoxicity	17, 18
Octreotide	Decreased CsA absorption	Decreased CsA concentrations	20, 21
Omeprazole	Increased CsA metabolism	Decreased CsA concentrations	1
Ranitidine	——	No effect	124–127
Nonsteroidal and other antiinflammatory agents			
Colchicine		Increased CsA concentrations with nephrotoxicity	121
Diclofenac	Decreased prostaglandin production	Increased nephrotoxicity	134
Indomethacin	Prostaglandin depletion	Increased nephrotoxicity	146
Sulfinpyrazone	Assay interference	Decreased CsA concentrations	1
Sulindac		Increased CsA concentrations	120
Sex hormones			
*Danazol	Decreased CsA metabolism	Increased CsA blood concentrations with nephrotoxicity	116
*Methyltestosterone	As above	Increased CsA blood concentrations with nephrotoxicity and hepatotoxicity	119
*Norethisterone	As above	Increased CsA blood concentrations with nephrotoxicity	116
Oral contraceptives	As above	As above	117, 118

Drug	Proposed Mechanism	Possible Effects	References
Steroids			
* Methylprednisolone	Unknown	Increased CsA plasma concentrations (RIA)	108
		Decreased CsA blood concentrations (HPLC)	109
		Convulsions	161,162
* Prednisolone	Competitive inhibition of cytochrome P-450	Reduced clearance and elevated prednisone concentrations	104–107
Miscellaneous			
Alcohol (heavy intake)	Decreased CsA metabolism Altered CsA absorption	Increased CsA concentrations	122
Atracurium	Unknown	Enhanced neuromuscular blockade (animal studies)	164
Doxorubicin	Unknown	Enhanced cytotoxicity	160
Etoposide	Unknown	Enhanced cytotoxicity	160
Fentanyl	Unknown	Enhanced analgesia (animal studies)	163
FK-506	Decreased CsA metabolism	Increased CsA concentrations and nephrotoxicity	49
* Melphalan	Unknown	Increased nephrotoxicity	135, 136
Metamizole	Unknown	Decreased CsA concentrations	1
Mizoribine	Unknown	Enhanced immunosuppression	160
Pentazocine	Unknown	Increased CsA concentrations	1
Tamoxifen	Unknown	Increased CsA concentrations	1
Vecuronium	Unknown	Enhanced neuromuscular blockade (animal studies)	164

* Substantiated interaction.
(Courtesy of Lake KD: *Pharmacotherapy* 11:110S–118S, 1991.)

Comments: Cyclosporine (CsA) has become a part of the immunosuppressive regimen for almost all types of patients with organ and tissue transplants. Although it has demonstrated value in preventing rejection of the transplanted tissue or organ, there are several complications related to CsA. Many of these complications are enhanced by drugs administered concomitantly with CsA. In addition, some drugs may decrease the immunosuppressive effectiveness of CsA and lead to a rejection episode. Thus, it is incumbent on every nurse who administers CsA to be aware of its potential side effects and interactions with other drugs.

This article should be on the reading list of every nurse who works with organ and tissue transplant recipients, especially critical care nurses who care for these patients during the immediate postoperative period when they are likely to be receiving multiple drugs. The table should be posted where it is conspicuous for every clinician who prescribes or administers drugs to organ and tissue transplant recipients. The references, which support the information in the table, would be worthwhile reading for the nurse who wishes to explore this topic in detail.—L.E. Lancaster, RN, MSN, EdD

Complications Associated With Immunosuppressive Therapy and Their Management

Min DI, Monaco AP (Northeastern Univ; Harvard Med School, Boston)
Pharmacotherapy 11:119S–125S, 1991 9–5

Problem.—Immunosuppression is associated with many general complications, including increased susceptibility to opportunistic infections or malignancy. In addition to these, particular immunosuppressive agents may be associated with specific side effects. Both the general and specific complications of immunosuppression are reviewed.

General Complications.—Transplant patients are prone to infection from all types of organisms, including bacteria, viruses, fungi, rickettsia, protozoa, and parasites. The signs may be subtle, and are often suppressed by the anti-inflammatory effects of the immunosuppressive therapy. Cytomegalovirus infection remains a problem, although high-dose

Specific Drug-Related Complications of Immunosuppressive Therapy

Drug	Complications	Management
Cyclosporine	Nephrotoxicity	1. Therapeutic drug monitoring to maintain CsA concentration within therapeutic range* 2. Protocol modification: sequential therapy: CSA initiation delays until 5–7 d or diuresis; conversion to AZA+P protocol after 3 mo posttransplant 3. Concurrent drug therapy: calcium-channel blockers (diltiazem, verapamil) thromboxane synthetase inhibitor
	Hyperkalemia	1. Diuretic therapy 2. Sodium polystyrene sulfonate 15-30 g with 30 ml of 70% sorbitol, if serum K^+>6 mEq/L
	Tremor	Dose reduction, if patient cannot tolerate it
	Hirsutism, gingival hyperplasia	Cosmetic treatment/careful dental hygiene
Azathioprine	Leukopenia, thrombocytopenia	Monitoring WBC and dose adjustment: 200 mg/day if WBC >10, 150 mg/day if 7.5 < WBC < 10, 100 mg/day if 5 < WBC < 7.5, 50 mg if 3.5 < WBC < 5, hold dose if WBC < 3.5
Corticosteroids	Adrenal suppression	1. After prolonged therapy, abrupt withdrawal may cause adrenal crisis. It should be tapered slowly. 2. Patient should carry identification card.
	Fluid and electrolyte disturbance	Diuretic therapy with close monitoring of electrolytes
	Cataracts	Regular eye examinations required
	Bone diseases	Regular bone examinations and if severe, surgical treatment
	Peptic ulcer	Adequate protection with antacid or H_2 blockers is necessary, especially with high doses
Polyclonal Antilymphocyte (antithymocyte) Globulin	Fever, chills	Acetaminophen 1300 mg p.o. and diphenhydramine 50 mg p.o. 30 min before dose
	Anaphylaxis	1. Before the first dose, skin test with 1 ml 1:1000 dilution P-ALG. 2. If patient develops anaphylactic reaction, stop infusion of P-ALG and epinephrine HCl s.c. or i.m. 0.2–0.5 mg (2–5 ml 1:10,000) with supportive care.
Monoclonal Antibody	First dose reaction	1 mg/kg methylprednisolone i.v. 2–6 hrs prior to the first dose and acetaminophen 1300 mg p.o. and diphenhydramine 50 mg p.o. 30 min before dose. 100 mg hydrocortisone i.v., 30 min after dose. If severe symptoms, meperidine 50–75 mg i.m. or i.v.
	Pulmonary edema	Careful check of patient's weight and if gains weight >3% during prior 7 d, wait until extra water is removed. If patient develops pulmonary insufficiency, supportive care with oxygen therapy and if necessary, intubate.
	Aseptic meningitis	Supportive care with symptomatic treatment with antipyretics and usually recover within 2–3 days even with continuation of OKT3. If patient has encephalitic symptoms, stop OKT3.

* Depending on analytic methods, sample matrix, and transplanted organ, therapeutic range may be different (i.e., high-performance liquid chromatography (whole blood) and polyclonal radioimmunoassay (whole blood) for kidney are 100–250 ng/mL and 400–800 ng/mL, respectively). (Courtesy of Min DI, Monaco AP: *Pharmacotherapy* 11:119S–125S, 1991.)

oral acyclovir and intravenous immunoglobulin therapy have shown some success. Immunosuppression may have to be reduced or even, for life-threatening infections, stopped temporarily to allow host defenses to work. Immunosuppressed patients also are at high risk for malignancies, especially lymphomas and skin cancers. Transplant patients have a mortality from hematologic malignancies 48 times higher than that of the general population.

Specific Complications.—The most serious complication of cyclosporine (CsA) is nephrotoxicity. This may be decreased by monitoring blood levels, modifying the protocol, or giving other agents along with CsA. Cyclosporine also may result in hepatotoxicity, hyperkalemia, hypertension, tremor, gingival hyperplasia, and hirsutism. Bone marrow suppression may occur in dose-related fashion in patients receiving azathioprine, often leading to leukopenia. Complete blood counts must be carefully monitored; adjusting the dose according to white blood cell count is usually sufficient.

Corticosteroids have many side effects, which cause the most trouble for patients who maintain their grafts for a long time. These may include slow healing and insulin-dependent diabetes mellitus. Many of these side effects decrease if the dosage is reduced or discontinued.

As foreign antibodies, the antilymphoblast and antithymocyte globulins may cause allergic-type reactions, including fever, chills, and hypotension. The initial side effects of monoclonal antibodies may be similar, with the addition of headache and rigors. Acetaminophen, antihistamines, and steroids may be given before injection to prevent this reaction. Monoclonal antibodies may cause pulmonary edema and are not given to patients who are gaining weight. Rarely, they cause aseptic meningitis or encephalopathy.

Conclusions.—The general and specific complications of immunosuppressants, including CsA, azathioprine, corticosteroids, polyclonal antilymphoblast and antithymocyte globulins, and monoclonal antibodies, are discussed. Strategies for management of some of the specific complications also are presented (table).

Comments: The management of transplant recipients presents the clinician with a major dilemma. The patient must be immunosuppressed to prevent rejection of the organ or tissue transplant, yet the immunosuppressive regimen almost always has dose-related minor to severe, life-threatening side effects. Thus, the clinician is constantly balancing the need for immunosuppression to maintain organ function against the potential complications of the specific immunosuppressants.

Although this article does not provide in-depth information about any one immunosuppressant, it does offer an excellent review of the most common complications of frequently used medications and their management. This review is excellent for the critical care nurse caring for the transplant recipient during the immediate postoperative period and, also, for the nurse who cares for these patients after hospital discharge and during lifetime follow-up. The table provides a synopsis of the most salient complications of frequently used agents and offers a quick review of their management. This table and the accompanying article should be readily available for reference to all members of the health care team who are involved in the care of organ and tissue transplant recipients.—L.E. Lancaster, RN, MSN, EdD

Transplantation's Newest Weapon: FK 506

Pezze JL, Whiteman K (Presbyterian Univ Hosp, Pittsburgh)
Am J Nurs 91:40–42, 1991 9–6

Background.—The experimental immunosuppressant FK 506 was first given in February 1989 to a transplant recipient facing rejection of her third liver in 3 years. The rejection process stopped during the next 2 weeks, and the patient eventually went home with a functional liver. The drug is a macrolide, a group of chemicals that originally became known for their antibacterial properties. After FK 506 was discovered, the group was studied for its immunosuppressant activity. Rapamycin is another member of this group with immunosuppressive properties. In August 1989 FK 506 was first given as primary therapy, prescribed before any other immunosuppressant. It has been used most often after liver transplants.

FK 506 Versus Cyclosporine.—Both drugs inhibit the cell-mediated immune response that "reads" the transplanted organ as foreign tissue to be destroyed, and both block the production of interleukin-2 and other lymphokines that help T lymphocytes proliferate. However, each drug suppresses T lymphocyte activation by binding to a different intracellular protein. Cyclosporine inhibits the phosphate-mediated release of calcium from mitochondria, and FK 506 does not. Although FK 506 is said to be 100 times more potent that cyclosporine, it seems to have less severe side effects. Its hepatotrophic effect, regenerating, repairing, and protecting liver cells, is also stronger.

Side Effects.—Side effects of intravenous infusion are nausea, headache, hyperesthesia, sensations of warmth, circumoral numbness and tingling, tremors, itching, flushing, abdominal pain, vomiting, and chest pain. Side effects are less common after oral dosing and include insomnia, headache, a "racing" sensation, tremors, and hair loss or hair growth. Most side effects disappear as the dose is reduced.

Conclusions.—Early clinical trials have shown that FK 506 prevents acute organ rejection with fewer overall side effects than with other immunosuppressants. In addition, it revives dying liver cells. Currently, FK 506 is under study for use in treating other immune disorders as well.

Comments: All posttransplant patients require an immunosuppressive regimen to prevent transplant rejection. Yet, the ideal immunosuppressant has not been developed. Currently, all immunosuppressive regimens are expensive and have numerous side effects. Many require that the patient remain in the hospital during administration of the medication. No wonder both transplant patients and health team members become excited when a new, less expensive immunosuppressive medication with fewer side effects than existing regimens becomes available. FK 506, which promises to be such a medication, currently is used only for liver transplant patients at the University of Pittsburgh. If it is successful in this patient population and if larger supplies can be obtained, it eventually will be used for other types of organ transplant recipients throughout the world. Because the immunosuppressive regimen begins immediately posttransplant in the critical care unit, nurses will be involved in administration and assessment of the patient's response to FK 506 therapy. Thus, nurses must be prepared to assume this responsibility. This short, but comprehensive, article provides basic guidelines for developing a protocol for FK 506 use. The information could be incorporated into a standardized nursing care plan and could be used as the basis for a continuing education session.—L.E. Lancaster, RN, MSN, EdD

10 Altered Skin Integrity

Classification of Nursing Interventions for Care of the Integument

Titler MG, Pettit D, Bulechek GM, McCloskey JC, Craft MJ, Cohen MZ, Crossley JD, Denehy JA, Glick OJ, Kruckeberg TW, Maas ML, Prophet CM, Tripp-Reimer T (Univ of Iowa, Iowa City)

Nurs Diagn 2:45–56, 1991 10–1

Problem.—A taxonomy of nursing interventions that will comprise all direct care activities that nurses perform for patients is being created by a Classification of Nursing Interventions research team. In phase I of this task, a list of intervention labels was created; in phase II, the labels are being systematically organized to build a taxonomy of nursing interventions. A study to validate interventions for nursing diagnoses related to the integument (i.e., impaired skin integrity, potential for impaired skin integrity, and altered oral mucous membranes) was reported.

Study Methods.—The study design was descriptive, using a 2-round Delphi technique to validate each of 12 interventions. The survey sample consisted of 29 skin care experts. The 12 labels were extracted (Table 1) from a large data base, and a definition, critical activities, and supporting activities were developed for each by using an adaptation of Fehring's model. The panel then rated how characteristic each activity was for a particular intervention on a Likert scale. After the second Delphi round, activities were weighted, and those with ratios of less than .50, corresponding to 3 on the Likert scale in terms of importance, were discarded as nonsupporting. Those between .50 and .80 were considered supporting activities. Those greater than .80 were labeled as major and were considered to be critical activities for the intervention. A total Intervention Content Validity (ICV) score was determined for each intervention.

Findings.—Skin surveillance received the highest ICV score, followed by bedrest care and pressure management. Activities for these 3 interventions, as well as for positioning, wound care (Table 2), and skin care-topical treatments were grouped together because they were appropriate for patients with actual or potential impaired skin integrity. The remaining interventions were grouped together because of their usefulness in treating actual and potential altered mucous membrane integrity and impaired skin integrity.

Nursing Implications.—Nursing activities essential to operationalize intervention labels for care of the integument were identified. These activities are appropriate for use in nursing information systems as well as in practice. Empirical evidence is provided that nurses agree about the

TABLE 1.—Twelve Skin Care Labels, Definitions, and Validity Scores

Intervention	Definition	ICV Score Round 1	ICV Score Round 2
Skin Surveillance	Ongoing monitoring of skin and mucous membrane integrity	.93	.88
Bedrest Care	Promotion of comfort, and safety, and prevention of complications for people unable to get out of bed	.79	.79
Pressure Management	Minimizing pressure to body parts	.67	.78
Positioning	Moving the patient or a part of the patient to provide comfort, reduce the risk of skin breakdown, promote skin integrity, and/or promote healing	.66	.77
Oral Health Maintenance	Maintenance and promotion of oral hygiene and dental health for patients at high risk for developing oral or dental lesions	.76	.77
Oral Health Restoration	Promotion of healing for patients who have oral mucosa or dental lesions	.75	.77
Wound Care	Prevention of wound complications and promotion of wound healing	.72	.76
Bathing	Cleaning of the body for the purposes of relaxation, cleanliness, and healing	.79	.75
Hair Care	Promotion of neat, clean, attractive hair	.64	.71
Nail Care	Promotion of clean, neat, attractive nails and prevention of skin lesions related to improper care of nails	.82	.70
Oral Health Promotion	Promotion of oral hygiene and dental care for patients with normal oral and dental health who are not at risk for developing lesions	.76	.69
Skin Care–Topical Treatments	Application of topical substances or manipulation of devices to promote skin integrity and minimize skin breakdown	.57	.66

Abbreviation: ICV, intervention content validity.
(Courtesy of Titler MG, Pettit D, Bulechek GM, et al: *Nurs Diagn* 2:45–56, 1991.)

activities they perform to carry out the interventions described at a conceptual level.

Comments: Stay tuned for future developments from these University of Iowa researchers. I would guess that we will see their research findings pre-

TABLE 2.—Wound Care

Definition: Prevention of wound complications and promotion of wound healing

	Weighted Ratio	
	Round 1	*Round 2*
Critical (Major) Activities †		
Provide incision site care.	.92	.83
Position to avoid placing tension on the wound.	.86	.84
Teach patient or family member(s) wound care procedures.	—*	.85
Maintain patency of any drainage tubes.	—	.88
Administer skin ulcer care.	.85	.89
Bandage appropriately.	.72	.89
Compare and record regularly changes in the wound.	—	.90
Inspect the wound with each dressing change.	—	.91
Note characteristics of any drainage.	.96	.91
Note characteristics of the wound.	—	.92
Supporting (Minor) Activities		
Massage the area around the wound to stimulate circulation.	—	.53
Shave the hair surrounding the affected area.	.53	.53
Clean with antibacterial soap.	.50	.53
Place affected area in a whirlpool bath.	.53	.55
Soak in saline solution.	.50	.57
Administer central venous line site care.	.72	.72
Apply an occlusive dressing.	.77	.72
Remove adhesive tape and debris.	.67	.72
Administer IV site care.	.78	.73
Administer Hickman line care.	.77	.73
Apply topical protectant to the affected area.	.52	.73
Dress with appropriate mesh gauze.	.73	.74
Apply an appropriate ointment to the skin/lesion.	—	.76
Maintain sterile dressing technique when doing wound care.	.91	.78
Reinforce the dressing.	.79	.78
INTERVENTION CONTENT VALIDITY SCORE	**.72**	**.76**

* Activities added after Round 1.
† Activities are worded as they were in Round 2 survey.
(Courtesy of Titler MG, Pettit D, Bulechek GM, et al: *Nurs Diagn* 2:45–56, 1991.)

sented in most major nursing journals and at most major nursing meetings in the future. Their work transcends specific patient care settings and applies to all of nursing practice because it is aimed at classifying nursing interventions for all treatment activities.

A nursing intervention is defined by the researchers as "any direct care treatment that a nurse performs on behalf of a client. Such treatments include nurse-initiated treatments resulting from nursing diagnoses, physician-initiated treatments resulting from medical diagnoses, and performance of the daily essential functions for the client who cannot do these." Thus, this definition includes all nursing activities and not just those independently performed by the nurse.

Identifying and classifying all interventions that nurses perform will provide a monumental breakthrough for nursing. From a handout by Titler at a National Teaching Institute presentation, I counted 312 different intervention labels that these researchers are investigating. This process will articulate what it is that nurses do and will clarify the unique activities of nursing specialty areas. For example, it will help to catalog what interventions nurses use in critical care to define the essence of critical care nursing practice. Moreover, the process will be used for costing out nursing services based on nursing diagnoses and their corresponding interventions. For example, we will be able to determine how much it costs to prevent skin breakdown, to do hemodynamic monitoring, to perform endotracheal suctioning, and to manage an artificial airway.

Because the activities that define a specific intervention will be validated, we will be able to use those lists to develop exemplary standards of care. For example, Table 2 demonstrates a validated list of critical activities necessary to carry out the nursing intervention of wound care. This list therefore provides the link between the nursing diagnosis of altered skin integrity and the desired patient outcomes (i.e., wound healing and preventing complications of altered skin integrity).

A complete list of all nursing interventions and their critical activities can be used to evaluate job performance and conduct quality assurance and patient outcome research (i.e., Are the critical activities being performed? Are they being performed properly? Are these activities achieving the desired patient outcomes?). In addition, based on a validated list of activities that define each nursing intervention, patient classification systems will be more highly refined based on sensitive criteria and patient care requirements. All of these advances will depend heavily on building an automated computerized nursing information system that ultimately could be used to identify a national data base to plan for resource allocation and to guide the direction of national health policy. The implications of this work are staggering. These researchers are to be congratulated.—C.E. Guzzetta, RN, PhD, FAAN

A Clinical Study of Hospital Replacement Mattresses

Johnson G, Daily C, Franciscus V (North Hills Passavant Hosp, Pittsburgh;

McKeesport Hosp, Penn; West Penn Hosp, Pittsburgh)
J Enterstomal Ther Nurs 18:153–157, 1991 10–2

Problem.—Pressure ulcers continue to be a serious problem. Hospital replacement mattresses (HRMs) may be described in advertising as "pressure-relieving" or "pressure-reducing"; these terms are not synonymous. According to the International Association for Enterstomal Therapy (IAET), a "pressure-relieving" device can consistently reduce pressure *below* the arterial capillary closing pressure of 25–32 mm Hg. A "pressure-reducing" device can reduce pressure down to 25–32 mm Hg. Studies of the levels of external pressure that can cause cell damage indicate that external pressure exceeding 20–40 mm Hg impedes blood flow in distal capillaries. This causes cell ischemia, a build-up of toxic cellular waste materials, detrimental histologic changes, and eventually cell necrosis. High levels of external pressure for a short time can be just as damaging as low levels for a longer time. The performance of a variety of HRMs in several hospitals was assessed.

Methods.—Fifty-five patients at 4 hospitals were assigned to 7 mattresses of different types. Risk assessment scores were calculated with a modified version of the Gosnell Risk Assessment Tool. Several factors were considered in the analysis but were not controlled: level of consciousness, nutritional status, continence, mobility, use of restraints, and diapers. Each patient's risk was scored to enable the selection of participants on the basis of their potential for pressure-ulcer development. Measurements were taken under the coccyx, trocanter, and 1 heel of all patients.

Findings.—The measuring device recorded a maximum reading of 100 mm Hg. Pressures greater than 100 were recorded as 100+ mm Hg. The pressures ranged from 24 mm Hg for 1 patient under the coccyx to 100+ mm Hg for 4 patients under the heel. The number of patients per mattress ranged from 5 to 17, with the average number of days of mattress use ranging from 5.5 to 11.8. Twenty patients already had ulcers before they were placed on the mattresses. Of the 30 stage I and II preexisting ulcers, 13 showed improvement, 3 deteriorated, and 14 did not change. Twenty new pressure ulcers developed. Nine were on the heels, 3 on the feet, 2 on the hips, 2 on the sacrum, 1 on the buttocks, 2 on the elbows, and 1 on the spine.

Nursing Implications.—According to the IAET definition of pressure relief—a reading of 32 mm Hg—none of the mattresses tested could be considered pressure-relieving. Institutions should consider eliminating the use of 2-inch foam mattresses. Higher quality overlays, such as static air mattresses, should be kept on hand until it is certain that the HRM chosen can adequately replace them. The use of higher quality overlays will probably decline with the increasing use of HRMs.

Comments: Beware of mattress representatives who claim their mattresses are pressure-relieving or pressure-reducing. This study demonstrated that 7 of the mattresses tested did not meet the criteria of the International Association of Enterstomal Therapy. Be an informed consumer of medical products. Request research data to support their claims or, better yet, perform your own studies before recommending the purchase of such mattresses. This is one of the strong points of this article.

Another point is the documentation of patients who developed pressure ulcers. Whereas there was improvement in the ulcers that existed at the beginning of the study, there were more ulcers that developed during the study, particularly on the heels. How do these numbers compare with the number of ulcers developed in your unit? The development of pressure ulcers has multiple contributing factors such as nutrition, tissue perfusion, degree of cortisol from stress, and patient age. Ulcers can be prevented, especially on the heels, by removing pressure and preventing shearing against bed linens. Prevention of ulcers can be simple and effortless, but is often overlooked. When this lack of prevention occurs and prolongs the patients' illness and/or hospitalization, we must assume some of the responsibility. Critical care nurses can make a difference in the outcomes of patients.—S.F. Wilson, RN, PhD

A Pilot Study of Interface Pressure With Heel Protectors Used for Pressure Reduction

Flemister BG (Mother Frances Hosp, Tyler, Tex)

J Enterstomal Ther Nurs 18:158–161, 1991 10–3

Problem.—Few investigations have focused exclusively on heel pressure. The incidence of heel ulcers reportedly was reduced through increased staff awareness of the problem and the use of a pressure-distributing material. Another report indicated that patients wearing socks in bed seemed less prone to sore heels. However, the traditional practice of applying heel protectors to patients at risk for pressure lesions is not supported by the literature.

Methods.—A pilot investigation was done to test the effectiveness of heel protector application in reducing interface heel tissue pressures. Seven patients who were at moderate-to-high risk for the development of pressure ulcers were examined. Pressure readings were taken under the heel. Polyester-based and foam heel protectors were tested and compared.

Findings.—The polyester-based heel protector had the highest pressure reading. The mean pressure of the support surface alone (mattress without heel protector) was 29.7 mm Hg; that of the foam heel protector on the support surface was 28.4 mm Hg; that of the polyester heel protector was 42.7 mm Hg. Thus, if patients are placed on a support surface, the high-density foam heel protector does not greatly reduce pressure. It slightly increased the interface pressures in 2 patients. Pressures generated with the polyester-material protectors were greater than those generated on the support surface alone in 6 of 7 patients and pressure was the same as that with the support surface alone in the seventh patient.

Nursing Implications.—The sample size in this investigation was very small; therefore, the results must be interpreted very cautiously. However, these findings suggest that pressure-reduction products may not adequately reduce pressure under the heels, indicating that current practices using heel protectors do not effectively eliminate the most important cause of ulcers—pressure.

Comments: Just as Abstract 10–2 alerted us that pressure-relieving mattresses do not relieve pressure, now we learn that heel protectors do not protect heels! Another nursing ritual has been challenged. Although this is only a pilot study with 2 styles of heel protectors used on only 7 patients, we should heed the warning. More research in this area is needed. Some hospitals use a mattress that is shorter than the bed frame so that the patient's heels actually hang off the end of the bed to protect them from pressure. Many times the foam booties are left in place until bath time, when the heels are inspected. Until more evidence is provided about the best way to protect heels from pressure, nurses must inspect the skin inside the heel protectors more often. Another way to react to the information in this article is to assess the severity of the problem. Determine the incidence of skin breakdown in your unit and the sites where this breakdown occurs. What types of heel protecting devices are you using and how effective are they? Request data from product representatives on the amount of pressure reduction that can be expected from specific products. In the roles of the patient advocate and informed consumer, we can make a critical difference in reducing hospitalization time and cost.—S.F. Wilson, RN, PhD

11 Pain

Intermittent Injection vs Patient-Controlled Analgesia for Sickle Cell Crisis Pain: Comparison in Patients in the Emergency Department
Gonzalez ER, Bahal N, Hansen LA, Ware D, Bull DS, Ornato JP, Lehman ME
(Med College of Virginia, Richmond)
Arch Intern Med 151:1373–1378, 1991 11–1

Problem.—Patients with sickle cell disease often are seen in the emergency department with acute pain from sickle cell crisis, and repeated administration of a parenteral narcotic often is necessary. Intermittent intravenous morphine injections were compared with patient-controlled analgesia (PCA) in patients seen in the emergency department with pain from sickle cell crisis.

Findings.—Use of PCA began sooner in the course of pain than did intermittent morphine injections. Pain scores did not differ substantially in the 2 treatment groups, nor did the total amounts of morphine administered, vital signs, or level of alertness differ significantly. Side effects (e.g., nausea, vomiting, pruritis) were comparable in the 2 groups. The PCA recipients had a shorter stay in the emergency department. Nurses rated PCA somewhat more favorably than the intermittent intravenous regimen, chiefly because of convenience and because patients were more involved with their care.

Nursing Implications.—The use of PCA is as effective a way of administering morphine to adult patients with sickle cell crisis as is a fixed-schedule regimen of intermittent intravenous injections.

Comments: The futurists for nursing are predicting that professionals will move away from a delivery system driven by needs of the system and toward a system driven by needs of the patients. Use of patient controlled analgesia (PCA) is an ideal strategy to accomplish this goal. Although the PCA pump requires more time to set up initially compared with the time required to prepare one injection, the time saving overall is considerable. Patients who value independence will appreciate being able to control their level of comfort while patients who prefer to be dependent may not value PCA. Studies of this kind need to be replicated with other and larger samples and in other nursing departments; however, the idea must not be lost. The use of PCA pumps provides a win-win-win situation: the patient can control the timing of analgesia, the nurse saves time, and the cost of the patient's stay may be shorter.—S.F. Wilson, RN, PhD

12 Altered Family Processes

Critical Care Nurse Perceptions of Family Needs

O'Malley P, Favaloro R, Anderson B, Anderson ML, Siewe S, Benson-Landau M, Deane D, Feeney J, Gmeiner J, Keefer N, Mains J, Riddle K (Miami Valley Hosp, Dayton, Ohio; Royal Children's Hospital, Melbourne, Australia)

Heart Lung 20:189–201, 1991 12–1

Problem.—Most previous research on family needs has centered on the family's perceptions when the patient is admitted to the intensive care unit (ICU) rather than on the nurse's perceptions, but there is an important relationship between the two. Perceptions of family needs by critical care nurses were studied.

Study Methods.—The sample was comprised of 126 nurses working in 4 ICUs in a large teaching hospital. During a 2-week period, the nurses were administered a "Needs of Families of Critically Ill Patients" questionnaire, a modification of Molter's "Needs of Relatives of Critically Ill Patients" questionnaire. This instrument addressed nurse's perceptions of the family's needs and of the time available to meet those needs. For needs identified as being best met by someone other than the nurse, respondents were asked who would be the best professional to meet those needs.

Findings.—Most of the respondents believed that the needs of the family were important or very important. Eighty-five percent of the nurses reported that they were capable of meeting these needs and had sufficient time to do so on a daily basis. The nurses ranked the family's cognitive needs as most important compared to their psychological, personal, or physical needs. Nurses working in the different units—coronary, medical-surgical, telemetry, and advanced care—rated needs differently, probably as a result of the patients' levels of acuity and lengths of stay. Perceptions of needs also were affected by units worked, length of time in nursing and critical care practice, and educational attainment.

Conclusions.—Most critical care nurses believed that family needs are important and that they have the ability and time to meet those needs. Their responses were affected by a variety of factors such as perceptions of importance, available time, treatment setting, and ability to meet the need. More study is needed, including a more refined questionnaire and assessments in differing institutions and geographic areas.

Comment: *See comment after Abstract 12–3.*

Critical Care Patients' Perceptions of Visits

Simpson T (Univ of Pennsylvania)

Heart Lung 20:681–688, 1991 12–2

Purpose.—Knowing patients' preferences for visits can assist the nurse in promoting a therapeutic social environment for recovery and in making clinical decisions regarding appropriate visiting policies. Visitation has been studied from the nurses' and families' perspectives, but patients' preferences for visiting have not been studied as extensively. The relationships among coronary care unit (CCU) and surgical intensive care unit (SICU) patients' preferences for visits and other personal and illness-related characteristics were examined.

Study Methods.—Fifty CCU and 50 SICU patients were verbally interviewed within 3 days of transfer from the unit to determine their preferences for visits, extraversion, age, socioeconomic status, physiologic and perceived illness severity, and evaluation of the helpfulness and fatigue associated with visits. The survey instruments included a questionnaire about patients' perceptions developed specifically for the study and reviewed by nurse researchers and the CCU and SICU head nurses. In addition, demographic characteristics, the Eysenck Personality Inventory, and the Acute Physiologic and Chronic Health Evaluation (APACHE II) classification system to measure illness severity were evaluated.

Findings.—The older the patient was, the longer the visit they preferred, particularly among CCU patients. Preferences for frequency of visits were similar to the patient's usual preferences for being with others. Patients' perceptions of their illness severity were positively related to the preferred number of visitors, particularly for SICU patients. A greater proportion of SICU patients than of CCU patients indicated that any time, day or night, was a good time for visits. Both groups mentioned afternoons as the best time period for visits and predominantly evaluated visits as helpful and not tiring.

Nursing Implications.—Knowledge about patients' preferences and evaluations of visits will provide insight for establishing appropriate visiting policies. Outcomes of interest to nurses include patients' anxiety levels after visits, the extent or occurrence of pain, and the impact of visits on patients' sleep or rest patterns. The diverse results of the patient survey suggest the importance of tailoring visits to patients' preferences and considering personal as well as illness-related characteristics.

Comment: *See comment after Abstract 12–3.*

Contracting for Visitation With Families

Moseley MJ, Jones A-M (Audie L Murphy Mem Veterans Hosp, San Antonio,

Tex; Med Ctr Hosp, San Antonio)
Dimens Crit Care Nurs 10:364–370, 1991 12–3

Purpose.—In the intensive care unit (ICU), visitation is an important aspect of patient care. As such, it should be part of the patient's care plan rather than at the discretion of the nurse. The importance and use of visitation contracts in the ICU were discussed.

The Visitation Contract.—When a visitation contract is used, visits are tailored to the family's needs to optimize the patient's support sources. Visits are predetermined, allowing the nurse to plan care around them. Liberalized visitation policies can have negative as well as positive effects for both patient and nurse. With visitation contracts, a balance can be struck between strict rules and nonstructured visitation.

Conditions of the Contract.—The patient's and family's visitation needs should be assessed as soon as possible after admission. Their preferences for visiting time, frequency, and duration are discussed. In completing the contract, the nurse assesses family dynamics, coping skills, and support levels. The contract then is included in the patient's care plan. One family member is identified as the contact person. This person is given daily reports and notified of any changes in the patient's condition to communicate to other family members. In the contracting process, a discussion of possible family roles may be engendered. Increasing the family's involvement in the patient's care may decrease their feelings of powerlessness. Patient care is structured around the family's and patient's needs. Contracting also allows family members to plan visits that are convenient to their own lifestyles. Signs should be posted that visiting hours are contracted. Visiting rooms must be close by and have telephones and food available.

Nursing Implications.—Contractual visitation is a helpful way to assess family needs, plan patient care, and base visitation on the family members' needs. As more patients are discharged early, it can also help family members identify which care-taking measures they can provide as they conserve their energy for the postdischarge period.

Comments: "To see or not to see". . . that is the question for many critical care nurses in determining when visitation can occur and who can visit. Along with ethical concerns and availability of supplies, patient families and visitation protocols are at the top of the list of "hot" issues for most critical care nurses. When dealing with families or setting visitation schedules, nurses wield enormous power. Decisions are often made based on assumptions, rituals, and tightly held values rather than family and patient needs.

Since Molter first studied the needs of family members of critically ill patients in 1979 (1), numerous other researchers have identified prioritized needs of the family. The research has relevance because the family is a vital link between the patient and society; not only does the patient's health affect the integrity of the family, but the family's health can profoundly influence patient recovery. Have research findings addressing family needs and visitation practices significantly changed nursing practice? Probably not to expected levels, as evidenced by the "we-they" attitude still held by many nurses toward families, and the restrictive, nonindividualized visiting hour policies still implemented in critical care units throughout the country. Perhaps family needs and visitation practices need to be explored from another angle to understand the problems better and to identify more workable strategies for change.

O'Malley et al. (Abstract 12–1) readjusted the research lens to focus on the nurses' perceptions of family needs. The resulting picture was found to be a little "out-of-focus." Whereas nurses did believe that family needs were important, they did not perceive family needs in the same priority as families perceived them. Thus, nurses were working with false assumptions. Family needs change over the course of hospitalization, first focusing on the need for hope and that hospital personnel cared about the patient. Later the need to know specific facts about treatment and that the best care was being given becomes a higher priority. Critical care nurses are often task-oriented. Thus, nurses answer questions, describe progress, and explain therapies that provide a less stressful avenue for interactions with families than discussions of subjective aspects such as grief, loss, and anxiety. This is especially so for the less experienced nurse. Perhaps more education in dealing with psychosocial issues would be beneficial as well as input by family members into patient care conferences and feedback from family satisfaction surveys.

Research has determined that more open and flexible visiting hours can impact both patient outcomes and family satisfaction positively. However, patients' feelings about visiting hours have not been aggressively explored until now. Results of Simpson's study (Abstract 12–2) provide insight for establishing beneficial visiting policies. Patients strongly value visitations, but with whom, when, and for how long varied with age, socioeconomic status, severity of somatic symptoms, personality type, and culture. Nurses need to assess patient's physiologic and psychological responses to visitation and adapt visitation schedules as necessary. For this to occur, a policy of flexible visiting hours is essential. To better individualize visiting hours based on patient and family needs, creative contracts for visitation may be developed, as suggested by Moseley and Jones in their informative, "how-to" article (Abstract 12–3). Such contracts would certainly allow more input by patient and family and help allay confusion about visitation "rules." If this strategy were used, would satisfaction levels of patients, families, and nurses improve? It is worth a try. We already know that current practice based on ritual and invalid assumptions doesn't work!—C. Kessler, RN, MN, CCRN, CS

Reference

1. Molter N: Needs of relatives of critically ill patients: A descriptive study. *Heart Lung* 8:332–339, 1979.

The Lived Experience of Survival and Bereavement Following the Death of a Lover From AIDS

Sowell RL, Bramlett MH, Gueldner SH, Gritzmacher D, Martin G (Med College of Georgia, Atlanta; Grady Mem Hosp, Atlanta; Univ of California, San Francisco)

Image: J Nurs Scholarship 23:89–94, 1991 12–4

Problem.—The death of a significant other is one of the most serious psychologic stressors a person can encounter. A special form of this stress occurs when a partner dies of complications of AIDS. In this setting the usual social support systems are lacking, and those affected are liable to remain isolated in their grief. Society at large is prone to disparage the significance of the relationship.

Study Methods.—Audiotaped interviews were conducted with 8 persons who had lost a partner to AIDS in the past 18 months. All subjects were men aged 26–53 years; 3 were health care professionals. In all instances but 1 the relationship had lasted longer than 3 years.

Findings.—Those who had lost their partner felt they were living only in a mechanical sense. They were isolated from relatives, friends, and themselves. Some had been reluctant to disclose their loss to any but their closest friends. A pattern of guilt, loneliness, anger, and ambivalence was frequently apparent and seemed to be more intense than the same feelings experienced by all those who grieve. A struggle to accept what had happened conflicted with the denial of loss.

Nursing Implications.—These findings are consistent with the mediators proposed in Sanders' theory of bereavement. They may be applicable to other settings where a significant other dies of a cause that is unacceptable to society. This may be death in an unpopular war such as Vietnam or a drug-related death. Nurses are challenged to develop interventions to facilitate effective resolution of grieving in this special group of patients.

Comments: No "tear-jerking" Hollywood production can do justice to the tragedy witnessed by nurses when a patient dies and the surviving loved-one plunges into the deep emotional abyss of grief. The energies recently placed on ministering to the dying patient now refocus on consoling the survivor, attempting to soothe the numbing despair many feel in the early phases of loss. The phases of bereavement and the needs of the survivor have been well researched and well known. Or have they?

This article argues that the surviving lover or life partner of an AIDS victim has unique concerns that are not sufficiently recognized by society or by the health care profession. With AIDS projected to become the second leading cause of death for individuals under sixty-five years old by the end of 1992 (1), and two-thirds of the AIDS cases involving homosexual transmission, an often hidden group of bereaved is emerging. Unlike other bereaved, the partners of AIDS victims often lack the customary support from family, bear the burden of social stigma associated with AIDS, and may have an additional fear of their own risk for developing AIDS. Thus, unsuccessful bereavement may be more likely.

Although the study reported here is hampered by several limitations, one of which is its small sample size (n=8), it provides moving testimonies from those surviving the death of a lover/partner from AIDS. Instead of a shoulder to cry on, many of these survivors receive society's cold shoulder, based on unsubstantiated fears and repressive values. Perhaps this, more than the death of their partner, is the real tragedy.—C. Kessler, RN, MN, CCRN, CS

Reference

1. Smith J, Stevenson L, Keeling R, et al: Everyday ethics in AIDS care. *AIDS Patient Care* 3:27–31, 1989.

Caregiver Issues

13 Ethical and Legal Issues

Demystifying Informed Consent
Cushing M (Salem, Mass)
Am J Nurs 91:17–19, 1991 13–1

Problem.—The involvement of nurses in informed consent ranges from witnessing a patient's signature on a form to explaining a procedure's risks and benefits and answering questions. Whatever the level of their involvement, nurses may worry about the legal risks of participation. Several issues related to informed consent are discussed.

Duty to Disclose.—Informed consent is the process by which a patient agrees to a procedure after a complete disclosure is made. The consent form documents that the disclosure has occurred. As a universal rule, the law recognizes that the physician is responsible for disclosure, not the institution in which treatment is given.

Nurse as Agent.—Nurses may act as physicians' agents in obtaining consent. In 1 court case, the law maintained that informed consent obtained by a nurse was acceptable when the information to be disclosed was within the scope of nursing practice. This court stated that the scope of information given to the patient was the most important consideration, rather than who provided that information.

The "Reasonable Person" Test.—A key concept in informed-consent cases is the "reasonable person" test. It must be shown that a reasonable person in his or her position would have consented to the procedure if informed properly.

Conclusion.—The best defense against legal problems with informed consent is preventing those problems in the first place. The best way to avoid such problems is to view disclosure not as a bureaucratic formality, but as an opportunity to inform and communicate with patients.

Comments: Informing and communicating with patients is a good defense against legal problems with informed consent; however, it is not sufficient. *Documenting* the information and communication also is necessary to avoid legal problems of any kind, including informed consent. Today we are seeking informed consent not only giving permission to perform care, but also giving permission to *withhold* care.

Clearly the physician has the duty to inform the patient and to determine whether the patient has understood the explanation. It is preferable for the defense of the physician in an informed consent case to have a member of the patient's family witness the explanation and sign the form as a witness (1). We have all observed physicians who either did not inform the patient sufficiently or who did so in a manner that the patient did not understand. Likewise we have witnessed patients who perhaps felt intimidated by the physician and stated an understanding of the physician's explanation and then confessed a lack of understanding to the nurse after the physician had left. Nurses thus have a responsibility to clarify information or answer questions when needed. Additionally we have the responsibility to inform the physician when patients revoke their consent. Patients have the right to change their minds about their consent. The American Nurses' Association's Code for Nurses with Interpretive Statements maintains that "whenever possible, clients should be fully involved in the planning and implementation of their own health. Each client has the moral right to determine what will be done with his/her person." Further, the Code directs nurses to protect consumers from misinformation and misrepresentation and to maintain the integrity of nursing (2). Patients must possess adequate information to enable an intelligent choice. The scope of communication must be measured by the information the individual patient needs to make a decision. The provider of this information should focus on the concerns of the patient (3). While reading Kelly, I also found this next quote of interest: "if the patient requests not to be informed of any risk, the provider has no duty to disclose (3)."

Our signatures as witnesses signify that the patient was the person who signed the permit. Our signature does not validate that the patient was informed. Our responsibility as a professional is to act as a patient advocate by educating patients so that they can make informed decisions about their bodies. This education is documented in the nurses' record and is authenticated with our signature.—S.F. Wilson, RN, PhD

References

1. Fiesta J: *The Law and Liability: A Guide for Nurses,* ed 2. New York, John Wiley & Sons, 1988, p 136.
2. American Nurses' Association: Code for Nurses with Interpretative Statements. Kansas City, Missouri, 1985.
3. Kelly ME: Informed consent, in Northrop CE, Kelly ME (eds): *Legal Issues in Nursing.* St. Louis, The C.V. Mosby Co, 1987, p 84.

Nurses' Perceptions of Powerlessness in Influencing Ethical Decisions

Erlen JA, Frost B (Univ of Pittsburgh)

West J Nurs Res 13:397–407, 1991 13–2

Problem.—An increasing emphasis has been placed on the ethics of nursing practice. Nurses' experience in influencing ethical decisions in patient care were examined. Specifically it addressed how nurses perceived their role when they were confronted with ethical dilemmas.

Study Methods.—In-depth interviews were conducted with 25 nurses directly involved in the clinical practice of nursing in an acute care setting over a 6-month period. The Perceptions of Nursing Ethics interview schedule was used.

Findings.—Three themes emerged from the interviews. The first was physician control, with the nurses seeing themselves as patient advocates. One nurse explained that because physicians had more power, physicians' wishes were carried out when their wishes conflicted with the patient's. When the nurses tried to intervene on the patient's behalf, physician control was again evident. The second theme was lack of knowledge of the alternatives. Some nurses expressed not knowing what the options were in certain situations. In a situation involving obtaining consent for coronary artery bypass surgery, 1 nurse stated that she did not know what steps to take for further action on the patient's behalf. The third theme was a nurse's ineffectiveness to influence the outcome or resolution of the dilemma faced. One nurse described a patient undergoing kidney transplant rejection who had a very poor prognosis and no will to live. However, the physicians were keeping the patient alive. This nurse said that everyone complained about the situation but no one did anything to remedy it.

Conclusions.—Nurses commonly expressed perceived powerlessness when there was physician dominance and a lack of knowledge about possible alternatives. When the nurses saw themselves as powerless, they described themselves as ineffective. Their inability to effect a resolution to a problem resulted in anger, frustration, and exhaustion.

Comments: The content analysis from interviews with 25 nurses revealed that they perceived themselves as powerless to effect ethical decisions involving patient care. So what else is new; many nurses feel this way. Nurses must move forward from the stage of ethical dilemma identification to actively participating in ethical dilemma resolution. The 3 themes identified in the study provide a beginning for nurses to learn to become more decisive in ethical issues. For example, in the situation of the physician who is too controlling, the nurse can consult with hospital resources such as other physicians, social workers, chaplains, and ethics committee members. Additional resources available are the Code of Ethics from the American Nurses' Association and the position statement from the American Association of Critical-Care Nurses. Call a meeting of these resource persons and the controlling physician so that diverse opinions can be discussed. Discuss with the controlling physicians the rationale they are using for their ethical decisions and ask that they listen to your rationale as well as those of the resource group.

The lack of knowledge about alternatives can be remedied by using the human and paper resources mentioned above. Also have discussions about hypothetical cases to learn about alternatives before an actual case. Create an algorithm of alternatives to use in different situations.

I believe that if the first 2 themes are resolved, then the third theme of ineffectiveness will be resolved. Nurses need to talk about their feelings in ethical issues with colleagues. This helps individual nurses articulate their personal beliefs and allows sharing among nurses. Each nurse can better understand his or her own beliefs by discussing them and, as a group, nurses can discover which nurses hold which beliefs. These beliefs must be respected, just as the patients' beliefs must be respected. The nurse must learn to separate personal beliefs from the beliefs of the patient when the two are in conflict. The role of patient advocate requires nurses to articulate the beliefs held by the patient even when they are in conflict with his or her own, or relinquish the role of advocate for this patient to another colleague.—S.F. Wilson, RN, PhD

The Challenge of Autonomy: Respecting the Patient's Wishes

Singleton KA, Dever R (Case Western Reserve Univ, Cleveland, Ohio; Fairview Gen Hosp, Cleveland)

Dimens Crit Care Nurs 10:160–168, 1991 13–3

Problem.—Critical care health professionals often deal with issues related to patient autonomy. Critical care nurses must be able to identify threats to autonomy and respond as patient advocates. A case that demonstrates autonomy issues facing many critical care patients was described.

Case Study.—Man, 67, underwent an emergency aortocoronary-bypass operation and was admitted to the intensive care unit. Just after surgery he required support of a left ventricular assist device. His course was unstable, and his prognosis was poor. Based on the patient's previously expressed wishes, his family asked that he not be resuscitated. They had no written evidence of his wishes, and the cardiothoracic team felt the request was premature. The team requested that all efforts for support be continued. The patient improved but remained dependent on mechanical ventilatory and hemodialysis support for 3 months. He was successfully weaned from the ventilator and recovered. He had full use of his mental capacities. His main wish was to go home. He was discharged, although still hemodialysis-dependent. A week later he was readmitted with acute pulmonary edema. The family requested no further mechanical support, including dialysis. Although the patient was fully alert and coherent, he was excluded from the discussion between his family and physicians. Physician's orders indicated no resuscitation and no dialysis. The patient recovered from this acute episode. He told his nurse he did not want "pounding" on his chest or the "tube" to breathe, but that dialysis made him feel better and was not too hard or tiring. The nurse relayed these comments to his physicians. A psychiatric assessment was done and found the patient competent to choose his own care. Hemodialysis continued until he died of cardiac arrest a few weeks later.

Conclusions.—The concept of autonomy includes independence, the right of reason to dominate in personal matters, and self-determination. The deontologic philosophical position supports this: persons have the right to determine what is and is not done to their bodies and to make decisions about their own lives. In the deontologic view, one is in complete control of one's own destiny and has the right to choose and follow one's own life plan. Quality of life can only be measured by the individual's own value system.

Nursing Implications.—Critical care nurses can play an important role by obtaining and documenting patient wishes for specific medical treatment, as illustrated in the case study. They can help determine whether patients have written or told others about such wishes and whether they have signed a Living Will or a Durable Power of Attorney. This information should be communicated to all those involved in the patient's care and placed in a prominent place in the patient's record.

Recommendations.—The following research questions are in need of further investigation:

- What assessment tool is reliable in measuring autonomy of acutely ill patients?
- How frequently do nursing admission assessment tools include questions about the patient's wishes for life-sustaining or life-maintaining measures?
- How frequently do nurses ask patients and family members whether the patient has signed a Living Will or Power of Attorney?
- What are the most common barriers to nurses responding as the patient's advocate?

Comments: Sometimes I forget that patients have a right to control their own destiny. Patients enter the health care system trusting that the health care team members will use their collaborative knowledge and skills to help patients regain their health. Once in the health care system, the patient is told when to eat, sleep, wake up, turn, cough, take medicine, sit up, lie down, and when family can visit. We take this control with the patients' permission and with their welfare foremost in our minds. For the patient who is unresponsive, we control their entire life.

Indeed it may be a challenge for us to respect the patient's wishes, especially when the patient's wishes are different from those we might choose if we were in a similar situation. The nurses' role as the patient advocate has evolved in this day of drugs and technology sophisticated enough to maintain life artificially. Advanced directives are useful in communicating patient's wishes; they allow patients to express their desires regarding life-sustaining treatment.

Nurses are in the most valuable position to know the patients' wishes and to help them manipulate the health care system to get what *they* want. The rationale for our actions comes from the American Nurses' Association's Code of Ethics, which mandates that nurses uphold the patient right of autonomy (1). In addition, the American Association of Critical-Care Nurses' position statement on patient advocacy is that critical care nurses are instrumental in providing an environment in which patient advocacy is expected and supported and that as a patient advocate, these nurses initiate and promote actions to promote the health care of the critically ill through social change (2). This change can occur within the hospital or within the community as we educate the consumer of health care about their rights.—S.F. Wilson, RN, PhD

References

1. American Nurses' Association: Code for nurses with interpretive statements. Kansas City, Missouri, 1985.
2. American Association of Critical-Care Nurses: Role of the critical care nurse as patient advocate. Aliso Viejo, California, 1989.

Legal and Ethical Implications of the *Cruzan* Decision for the Elderly, Their Families, and Health Care Providers

Spielman B, Fletcher JC (Univ of Virginia, Charlottesville)
Fam Community Health 14:81–88, 1991 13–4

Introduction.—The Supreme Court in *Cruzan v Missouri Department of Health* held that, although a competent person has the constitutionally protected right to refuse life-sustaining treatment including artificial nutrition and hydration, states may require clear and convincing evidence of an incompetent patient's desire to withdraw life-sustaining treatment and may choose to ignore the substituted judgment of close family members in the absence of substantial evidence that their views reflect those of the patient.

Consequences.—The Cruzan case constitutionalized a competent patient's right to die. Thus, competent adult patients cannot be forced to undergo medical treatment against their wishes. Three states have adopted stringent standards of proof for the clear and convincing evidence rule. Incompetent patients must have a previously executed living will or durable power of attorney. The state can constitutionally foreclose the option of private decision-making between health care providers and families.

Options.—All adults, their families, and their health care providers can document patients' wishes in such a manner that the documentation will hold up in a state that enforces the clear and convincing evidence rule. All 50 states and the District of Columbia have general durable power of attorney statutes that allow a person to designate a surrogate decision maker. Sixteen states and the District of Columbia permit surrogate decisions on life-sustaining treatment, even for patients who are not terminally ill. Ten states allow surrogate medical decisions, but only for terminally ill patients.

Documentation.—A patient's medical preferences may be documented from conversations between a professional and a patient or from structured interviews. Forty-four states and the District of Columbia have living-will laws that permit terminally ill patients who are still capable of decision-making to specify which treatments they wish to forego. Effective November 1991, the Patient Self-Determination Act requires Medicare and Medicaid providers to inform all patients about their rights under state law to execute living wills and durable powers of attorney. When conflicts arise after admission to a health care facility, an ethics committee may be consulted that may help identify the problems, discuss them with relevant decision makers, and attempt to mediate the dispute.

Conclusion.—The Cruzan decision allows adults to protect their interests by carefully documenting their desires and exercising informed choice when seeking health care.

Comments: Whereas this article describes implications of the Cruzan decision for the elderly, the implications are applicable to all persons. The message for critical care nurses is that we have a role as a patient advocate in the clinical setting in addition to an education role in the community. In the clinical setting, critical care nurses have a responsibility to carry out the wishes of the patient as described in their living wills or as indicated by a representative acting on their behalf through a durable power of attorney. If the patient wants all life-sustaining treatment possible, then this is the view of the nurse advocates with others: nurses, physicians, team members, and family; whether the nurses agrees with this view or not.

Conversely, if a patient wants all life-sustaining treatment withdrawn, including nutrition and hydration, they have the legal right to do so, provided they were competent at the time of request, have a living will stating their requests, or have a person acting on their behalf through a durable power of attorney.

The community role of the critical care nurse is to educate people about living wills and durable powers of attorney. This can be an individual effort by speaking to community groups, or a group effort such as through a local chapter of American Association of Critical-Care Nurses by providing information at health fairs and fun runs.

Critical care nurses are practicing in an environment where patients are more informed about their rights and some physicians are unwilling to relinquish their controlling power. This situation places the nurse between these 2 forces in the patient advocacy role.—S.F. Wilson, RN, PhD

Amyotrophic Lateral Sclerosis and Life-Sustaining Therapy: Patients' Desires for Information, Participation in Decision Making, and Life-Sustaining Therapy

Silverstein MD, Stocking CB, Antel JP, Beckwith J, Roos RP, Siegler M (Univ of Chicago; Montreal Neurological Inst)

Mayo Clin Proc 66:906–913, 1991 13–5

Problem.—Weakness in patients with amyotrophic lateral sclerosis (ALS) progresses gradually, resulting in a long clinical course. Thus, patients and their families have time to think about the disease and to discuss their feelings and thoughts with each other and with health care providers. Therefore, patients with ALS have the opportunity to make informed decisions in advance about life-sustaining treatment interventions. A longitudinal investigation was conducted to learn more about the wishes of patients with ALS for information about their disease and for intensive end-of-life care.

Patient Privacy.—Of 38 patients interviewed, 37% (14 patients) said they usually were seen alone by a physician when they came to the clinic. The other 63% (24 patients) usually were accompanied by a relative; these patients tended to have more advanced disease. Of these 24, 38% said they would like to consult with their physician alone.

Wish to Participate in Decisions.—Seventy percent (26) of the 38 patients questioned said that they preferred to participate in decisions about their own medical care. The rest preferred to leave those decisions to the physician.

Life-Sustaining Care.—Forty-seven percent (18 patients) said they had talked to someone about their wishes for life-sustaining care in extreme situations. Most had spoken with a spouse. Although only 8 of the 18 had talked with their physician, 81% said they thought their physician wanted to know their preferences about life-sustaining treatment. Half of the patients said they would like to discuss life-sustaining treatment with someone at the clinic. Of these, 10 wanted the physician to broach the subject. When asked about their wishes in different hypothetical situations, the patients' responses sometimes changed with time. Some patients changed their minds from not wanting to wanting resuscitation, and others decided they no longer wanted to be resuscitated.

Conclusions.—Discussions about ventilator support, intubation, and resuscitation should be initiated with patients with ALS who desire such conversations. Because patient preferences may change over time, a single discussion about cardiopulmonary resuscitation, ventilator support, or the writing of a living will may be inadequate to determine a patient's intentions. Patient wishes should be reevaluated throughout the course of the illness.

Comments: Amyotrophic lateral sclerosis (Lou Gehrig's disease) is a neuromuscular disease that eventually results in the paralysis of all muscles except a few of the cranial nerves and usually leads to death in 2 to 6 years after diagnosis. Reading this article had a great impact on me for several reasons. Although the sample size was small (N = 38) and the study needs to be replicated, it has a message for critical care nurses. I was impressed by the fact that some of the patients with ALS changed their minds from *not wanting* resuscitation to *wanting* resuscitation during a 6-month period. The patients I have known who had decided on no resuscitation either had not changed their minds or had made the decision very close to the time of their death. What we can learn from this article is the need to verify with patients that they still want to abide by the terms of their earlier decisions and living wills.

Another interesting fact was that 11 of the 38 patients did not want to participate in decisions about their health care. They preferred to leave these decisions to the physician. Nevertheless, I believe we have a responsibility to lay out the options for these people anyway and allow them at least the opportunity to make their own decisions.

Patient privacy is another interesting issue. Nine of the 24 patients who saw the physician with a family member would have preferred to see the physician alone. Perhaps if the patient is unable to request time alone with the physician, we could create the opportunity for them by arranging for the physician to see the patient alone first. Likewise, when talking to patients about their care, I usually make the assumption that the family should be involved. Now I am going to verify this assumption with the patient.

We can learn a great deal by listening to our patients. Incorporating their ideas and wishes make us more effective in our practice.—S.F. Wilson, RN, PhD

Neurologic Syndromes and Prolonged Survival: When Can Artificial Nutrition and Hydration be Forgone?
Cranford RE
Law Med Health Care 19:13–22, 1991 13–6

Purpose.—This paper addresses the question of under what medical conditions does it become ethically appropriate to withdraw (or withhold) artificial fluid and nutrition. The question applies to patients whose disease is so overwhelming that death is expected in a relatively short time whether or not medical treatment continues. It also applies to those with severe, irreversible illness or disablement who nevertheless may live for some time.

Criteria for Withholding Support.—Few disagree with not starting nutrition and hydration in a patient whose death is imminent. For the second category of patients, support should not be limited unless the ability to eat and drink normally has been lost, and unless the patient's disease is substantially and irreversibly disabling. The most common disabling neurologic conditions compatible with prolonged survival are persistent vegetative state, dementia, and severe, permanent paralysis. In many of these patients, there is a disparity between preserved vegetative functions and the loss of those functions that make us uniquely human: thinking, feeling, interacting with others. Affected patients can survive for some time if given aggressive medical treatment.

Outcome.—Patients in vegetative state usually die within 1–2 weeks of stopping nutrition and hydration. They die not of starvation but of acute dehydration. Survival for longer than 4 weeks suggests that someone is surreptitiously feeding or hydrating the patient.

Conclusion.—If support is to be withdrawn, suffering can be prevented by adequate doses of morphine, sedatives, analgesics, or hypnotics. Even if a patient were capable of suffering, the suffering that would inevitably take place during months or years of ongoing support must be taken into account. Today families are more likely to request that artificial nutrition and hydration not be started.

Comments: One resource nurses have for making ethical decisions is the American Nurses' Association (ANA). Guidelines on Withdrawing or Withholding Food and Fluid identify the ethically apparent reasons for giving or withholding food and fluid. "First, nurses should almost always provide food and fluid because it is almost always an essential, life-preserving, health-giving benefit. Second, nurses should temporarily withhold food and fluids when their very provision clearly causes harm (1)." An example of this latter guideline is withholding food and fluid from the preoperative patient or the infant with tracheoesophageal fistula. The conflict develops when we are not sure whether food and fluid are beneficial or harmful. "Withholding of food and fluids might be indicated only when feeding is futile because of underlying incorrectable absorption problems; when it is itself burdensome to the patient or sustains life only long enough to die of other more painful causes (1)."

An argument for maintaining feeding and hydration for patients is that it will prevent suffering associated with starvation and dehydration. One view I have heard is that when care rendered by a physician in a hospital is withheld or not initiated, then care rendered by a mother at home should be maintained (e.g., food, fluids, and comfort). Cranford points out, however, that persons who have experienced brain death or are in a persistent vegetative state are incapable for perceiving suffering. They experience no physical or psychologic suffering. One can justify withholding food and fluids based on the fact that these patients die in 1–2 weeks. Once the decision is made to withhold treatment together with feeding and hydration, the patient can be moved out of the ICU because treatment and close monitoring are no longer necessary. What care is required then for these patients during their last week or two of life? What care would you want your family member to have in this situation? Death is a part of the life process, and despite all the technology and treatment advances, we cannot keep all people alive. These individuals deserve a peaceful death. This includes maintaining their cleanliness and comfort as well as touching them and talking to them. Family members may choose to assist in providing this care as they say good-bye.—S.F. Wilson, RN, PhD

Reference

1. American Nurses' Association Committee on Ethics: Guidelines on withdrawing or withholding food and fluids. Kansas City, Missouri, 1987, pp 1–2.

14 Critical Care Environment

Guidelines for Categorization of Services for the Critically Ill Patient
Task Force on Guidelines of the Society of Critical Care Medicine
Crit Care Med 19:279–285, 1991 14–1

Purpose.—The Task Force on Guidelines of the Society of Critical Care Medicine presented the Guidelines for Categorization of Services for the Critically Ill Patient.

Levels of Care.—Two levels of care were outlined. Level I units deliver care to the desperately ill patient with complicated needs that require the continuous availability of sophisticated equipment, specialized nurses, and physicians trained in the care of critically ill patients. Level IC units deliver this high level of care; level IA units have an additional commitment to education and research in the field of critical care medicine and nursing. Level II units are found in hospitals that serve communities with limited resources. Although these centers often may be able to deliver high quality care to patients with single-organ failure, patients with complicated needs or multisystem organ failure must be transferred. Cooperative protocols will be developed between level II and Level I units relating to the care of the desperately ill during stabilization and transport. Standards for level II units are minimal standards for critical care units.

Implications.—Cooperation among hospitals and professionals in the same region is essential to ensure that an appropriate number of level I and level II units are designated. Redundancy would lead to poor use of resources, inability to maintain skills, and lack of cost-effectiveness. State and federal governments should be encouraged to implement reimbursement schedules that acknowledge the high cost of caring for the critically ill.

Comments: These are important statements from the Society of Critical Care Medicine (SCCM) regarding basic requirements (and philosophy) of how intensive care units (ICUs) should be operated and equipped. Included in these statements is a designation of the types of units that are present in a community. Through these statements, SCCM supports the role of nursing in the critical care team (although it is disappointing no nurses were listed as being on the task force). Several interesting nursing recommendations are present, such as the manager of the ICU not only having certification but also having

ICU experience. This runs counter to some administrator's philosophy that any manager can run any type of unit. Also, basic equipment and support services are listed, which may be of value to any unit uncertain about having appropriate technical equipment. Nurses should be aware that the equipment listed as necessary is usually present in any ICU, but not always. For example, end tidal Co_2 (Pet Co_2) monitors may not be available in all units. This is potentially important from both a quality of care and legal perspective.

Nursing needs to work closely with professional organizations interested in critical care. The SCCM traditionally has been a good colleague to the American Association of Critical-Care Nurses (AACN) in supporting goals in critical care. This document reflects that continued collegial relationship. Statements such as this from SCCM hopefully would lead to joint position statements from organizations such as AACN (something that has been done in the past). By using a multidisciplinary approach to standards, it is more likely to improve the type of care delivered to patients in the critical care setting.—T. Ahrens, RN, DNS, CCRN

Patterns of Resource Consumption in Medical Intensive Care
Oye RK, Bellamy PE (Univ of California, Los Angeles)
Chest 99:685–689, 1991 14–2

Problem.—As intensive care units (ICUs) have increased in number, their charges have increased to 20% of total hospital charges. Most reports show underreimbursement for intensive care under the prospective payment system, but there may be some patients for whom intensive care is probably not indicated and whose hospital charges are therefore inflated. Patterns of consumption of ICU resources, including the proportions of those resources used by patients admitted for monitoring only, were examined.

Methods.—A group of 404 consecutive medical ICU admissions to a university medical center during a 7-month period was examined. A utilization review nurse totaled therapeutic intervention scoring system (TISS) points for each patient on each day to estimate consumption of resources. There were 356 different patients (mean age, 55.7 years). Median ICU stay was 3 days, and in-hospital survival was 83%.

Findings.—Median resource consumption per admission, expressed as the sum of TISS points for ICU days, was 36; mean resource consumption was 113. The admissions with the highest 8% of TISS points consumed about half of the total ICU resources used. These "high-cost" patients had more chronic illness, more severe illness, more intense care, more do-not-resuscitate orders, and reduced survival rates. The "low-cost" patients included all patients admitted for monitoring only, and they consumed less than one tenth of the total resources.

Conclusions.—There is a skewed distribution of resource consumption in the ICU, with a minority of high-cost patients using a disproportionate amount of resources. Charges would be affected little by cutting back on the number of patients admitted for monitoring only. Mortality is high in high-cost patients; resource expenditures might be reduced by improved understanding of prognosis and better communication between the patient and physician.

Comments: This article addresses an important consideration in critical care resource use. The authors point out an observation that many of us who work in the ICU setting probably inherently already know; that is, many of the most critically ill patients, the ones most likely to die, are also the ones that consume the most resources. While the data from the study is older (collected in 1984 and 1985), it is probably still valid and corroborates what has been found in other studies. More interesting than the study data though, is one of the authors' recommendations. They state the discussion of diagnosis, prognosis, and likelihood of benefit might enlighten the patient and family regarding decisions of how to proceed with treatment. The key issues here are informed understanding and good communication. In this area, nurses play a vital role. Ensuring patient and family understanding of likelihood of benefit from therapy is more likely to fall to the primary and associate nurses because of the relationship that develops during the ICU stay.

The ethical issues of this study are important, with a clear implication that ICU use can be controlled effectively through informed patients and families self-limiting treatment options. If this implication is true, particularly in light of advance directives, resource use will decrease. However, for patients and family to self-limit therapies, a considerable improvement in communication from nurses and physicians will be required. This is one of the greatest challenges of the 1990s in health care.—T. Ahrens, RN, DNS, CCRN

15 Professional Issues and Trends

Use of Listening Skills When Advising Nursing Students in Clinical Experiences

Edwards EJ (Indiana Univ, Pennsylvania, Indiana, Pa)
J Nurs Educ 30:328–329, 1991 15–1

Problem.—Nurse educators often have difficulties advising nursing students during clinical experiences. When the instructor and student meet to evaluate clinical skills, the situation may be tense. Students' anxiety may hinder their learning. Listening skills can be used to facilitate communication in these situations.

Listening Skills.—Listening is often thought of as a passive process; however, good listeners are very active. Instructors must ensure that they understand what the student is saying and that they receive and respond to the whole content. Instructors help students talk about all the parts of their concern, not just the superficial or immediate aspects. Instructors also should be responsive in such a way that students experience being attended to and know that they have been heard.

Paraphrasing.—The most basic listening skill is paraphrasing. Instructors repeat the message in their own words, possibly using a concrete illustration, example, or metaphor. Paraphrasing involves summarizing whole units of the student's behavior, mirroring the student's thoughts, feelings, and actions. Paraphrasing allows the student to correct any misinterpretations that the instructor might have had.

Perception Check.—A perception check clarifies what the student has said. The instructor makes inferences and requests feedback on the accuracy of those inferences.

Summaries.—After the student has talked for a while, certain patterns may emerge that can be referred to as themes. Summarizing those patterns and themes allows instructors to check their understanding of the situation and to encourage students to explore their ideas more completely.

I-Statements.—These statements reflect the instructor's feelings, thoughts, or behaviors rather than what is felt about the student. One such remark is, "I feel uncomfortable telling you what to do." Beginning statements with "I" places the responsibility with the instructor, rather than the student. A statement such as, "That remark is confusing," places the responsibility with the student for the instructor's feelings and is unhelpful. I-statements are effective when they are combined with a perception check or paraphrase.

Conclusions.—Good listening is an active process. Meaningful listeners use a variety of specific listening skills and techniques to ensure that the student is heard and understood. These techniques include paraphrasing, perception checks, summarization, and I-statements.

Comments: Don't bypass this abstract just because you are not a student or a clinical instructor. This article is about listening and responding to others regardless of your role. Even if we assume we are good listeners, we can judge our skills against the ideal standard described in this article.

Critical care nurses use listening skills daily in interacting with patients, family members, nurses, other health care team members, and hospital managers. Think of the many ways you can apply this content! When explaining procedures or teaching patients and families, ask them to repeat what you have said. The nurse can *paraphrase* family member feelings, (e.g., "It sounds like you are blaming yourself for your son's accident). *Perception checks* are essential when listening to a colleague describe an incident (e.g., "As you describe all the demands on your time and energy, I have an image of someone with ropes tied to all parts of the body and people pulling these ropes in all directions at once. Is that how you feel?"). *Summarizing* what has been said is important after teaching patients and families, patient care conferences, and employee conferences. The *I-statement* is valuable to reflect back to the other person the feelings you have developed while they were talking (e.g., "As I listen to your description, I find myself getting very tense and tight. Is that what is happening to you?"). Try these strategies and notice the positive differences.—S.F. Wilson, RN, PhD

The Merit and Significance of Cinical Nurse Specialists

Boyd NJ, Stasiowski SA, Catoe PT, Wells PR, Stahl BM, Judson E, Hartman AL, Lander JH (Richland Mem Hosp, Columbia, SC)

J Nurs Adm 21:35–43, 1991 15–2

Problem.—It has been assumed that the clinical nurse specialist, a masters-prepared nurse, could merge the roles of clinician, educator, and scholar. A pilot investigation found that the nurse specialist was able to merge the clinician and educator roles but was less able to integrate the role of scholar. A 2-year follow-up to this previous investigation was done to further assess the merit of the clinical nurse specialist role.

Methods.—This descriptive investigation included 26 clinical nurse specialists at 1 institution. The clinical nurse specialist's job description was reviewed. Role was defined as to both the expected and actual behaviors.

Findings.—These clinical nurse specialists were able to merge and implement the roles of practitioner, educator, scholar, and consultant, as outlined in their job descriptions. The greatest amount of these nurses' time (47%) was spent in the practitioner role. However, they also spent 25% of their time as educators, 10% as scholars, and 8% as consultants. The nurses had published papers and produced revenue through grant proposals. Paradigm cases revealed that the clinical nurse specialists had a positive impact on patient care outcomes. The significance of the clinical nurse specialist role was documented by the outcomes of weekend coverage, serious occurrence reviews, and clinical logs.

Nursing Implications.—These findings indicate that hiring clinical nurse specialists who can efficiently combine these 4 important roles is a good investment. The support of nurse executives, who make budgetary decisions, is vital to the introduction and implementation of the clinical nurse specialist role in an institution. The value of this position should increase in the future, as budgetary pressures intensify and issues of supply and use of labor and productivity become more important.

Comments: One of the most perplexing role issues in nursing is the value of clinical nurse specialists (CNSs). This issue is vital to nursing because the CNS is the terminal level for advanced clinical practice. If the CNS role is not present, nursing has no system in place to develop expert clinical practice.

The issue of whether the CNS's salary can be justified to administrators is controversial. No major national study has been performed that addresses this issue. Without national studies to answer the CNS value question, CNSs across the country frequently report on empirical evidence in support of their position. Interestingly, no papers have been written that dispute the value of the CNS. In this paper, the authors do a good job of addressing some of the overt values of the CNS position. The methods of demonstrating value are valid and objectively measureable. Their results are consistent with other empirical literature on the topic. While some parts of their study may not demonstrate optimal use of the CNS role, (e.g., weekend supervisory coverage and no evaluation addressing the direct impact of advanced practice on patient outcome), the authors do outline the value that CNSs provide to an organization.

Clearly a national, prospective, randomized study is necessary to address the value of the CNS more completely. However, empirical evidence such as provided in this paper is consistent in supporting the role. Administrators would be wise to evaluate the use of CNSs for many reasons, ranging from improving clinical practice and patient outcomes to addressing specific clinical issues facing hospital and nursing administration.—T. Ahrens, RN, DNS, CCRN

Competence Statements for Differentiated Nursing Practice in Critical Care

Hickey M, Billings DM, Disch J, Eagleton B, Farrell MC, Turzan L, Vitello JM
(American Assoc of Critical Care Nurses Competency Task Force)
Focus Crit Care 18:286–293, 1991 15–3

Purpose.—The American Association of Critical-Care Nurses (AACN) has developed competence statements for differentiated nursing practice in critical care to provide a framework for health care agencies, nurse educators, managers, and researchers who wish to explore the possibility of implementing differentiated practice. Differentiated nursing practice, the process used in developing the AACN's competence statements, and potential uses of the AACN statements were examined.

Developing the Competence Statements.—Consultation and a review of the literature were the first step in generating competence statements. Second, terms to be used were operationally defined. "Differentiated practice" was defined as the 2 levels for nursing practice based on educational preparation—the baccalaureate and associate degrees. "Competence statements" are broad descriptors of nurses' behaviors—cognitive, affective, and psychomotor—that can be assessed and that differentiate the categories of nursing practice. The third step was to develop the statements that differentiate professional and technical critical care nursing practice (table). The last step was the validation of competence statements.

Potential Uses of Competence Statements.—In clinical practice, the statements could be used to assist in determining appropriate patient care assignments and in defining more realistic position and role expectations. In management, the statements could be used to develop position descriptions, to develop criteria for performance evaluations, and to correlate nursing salary ranges. The statements could be used in curriculum development or continuing education in nursing education. These statements could also be useful in research and legislative arenas.

Nursing Implications.—The AACN developed these competence statements to address specific behavior that reflects the valuable contributions of each category of nurses in critical care. They provide a model for efficient, effective practice patterns that may enhance the quality of outcomes of critically ill patients and their families.

Comments: This is an important philosophical document from the American Association of Critical-Care Nurses (AACN) addressing the controversial issue of differentiated practice. The authors address why the AACN believes in differentiated practice and describe the process for developing the statements (table), which describe the difference between 2 levels of nurses, the "Professional Nurse" and the "Associate Nurse." This is an admirable attempt by a major nursing organization to clarify the potential difference in education between nurses and how this might impact critical care.

Competence Statement Examples

Role Component: Clinical Practice

"Professional Nurse"

1. The professional nurse organizes and analyzes data to determine patient problems and to determine and formulate nursing diagnoses.

"Associate Nurse"

1. The associate nurse organizes and analyzes data to determine well-defined patient problems and to select nursing diagnoses from an established list.

Role Component: Management

"Professional Nurse"

1. The professional nurse implements and modifies delivery systems for nursing care that promote quality and efficiency of critical care nursing practice.

"Associate Nurse"

1. The associate nurse provides care consistent with the established delivery system for nursing care.

Role Component: Teaching

"Professional Nurse"

1. The professional nurse designs, implements, and evaluates a comprehensive teaching plan.

"Associate Nurse"

1. The associate nurse implements and individualizes standard teaching plans.

Role Component: Research

"Professional Nurse"

1. The professional nurse integrates research findings into critical care nursing practice.

"Associate Nurse"

1. The associate nurse uses research-based procedures in providing patient care.

Role Component: Consultation

"Professional Nurse"

1. The professional nurse serves as a resource in his or her area of practice.

"Associate Nurse"

1. The associate nurse seeks assistance from the professional nurse regarding issues of clinical practice.

Note: A complete listing of competence statements can be found in AACN's *Competence Statements for Differentiated Nursing Practice in Critical Care*. Newport Beach, California: American Association of Critical-Care Nurses, 1989.

(Courtesy of Hickey M, Billings DM, Disch J, et al: *Focus Crit Care* 18:286–293, 1991.)

It is also crucial to keep in mind, however, that until education changes to the point that actual measureable differences exist between graduates of different programs (e.g., associate and baccalaureate), this concept will be highly controversial. The AACN has taken a practical approach in this matter, indicating the uses of this document may be appropriate for some (where legislation has already been developed requiring a difference in practice) and not appropriate or timely for others. Although the key to nursing coming together over this issue is the production of truly different nurses in regard to capabilities, this key does not appear to be available for the immediate future. As such, expect controversy in this area for the rest of this decade. Unfortunately, this controversy does not help nursing achieve a cohesiveness that is essential in this volatile era of health care.—T. Ahrens, RN, DNS, CCRN

A National Board for Nursing Certification

Hartshorn JC (Univ of Texas, San Antonio)

Nurs Outlook 39:226–229, 1991 15–4

Introduction.—Nurses have long sought certification as a means of signifying their competence in special areas of practice. Certification programs have burgeoned in response, all with their own different standards. An initiative to create national standards for nursing certification was proposed.

Problems.—As graduate nurses begin to practice, they soon find they are unprepared for practice in their chosen specialty area. Some gain specialized knowledge through experience, continuing education, or self education, and they seek certification to demonstrate this nursing expertise. For nurses demonstrating proficiency, certification demonstrates competence and confers respect. However, there are now more than 30 organizations offering certification and nearly twice as many ways of achieving it. Nearly 200,000 nurses may have achieved certification, but standards vary to the extent that "certification" has no consistent meaning within nursing. Health care consumers may find the concept confusing. Specialty certification can improve nursing practice only after nurses, employers, regulatory agencies, and consumers recognize the meaning and importance of these credentials.

American Board of Nursing Specialties.—In response to these problems, 8 national nursing organizations banded together to form the American Board of Nursing Specialties. These organizations represent more than 120,000 certified nurses, comprising more than 65% of currently certified registered nurses. Sound organizational working principles have been established (table) and are well accepted, although there is controversy over the requirement for baccalaureate preparation.

Working Principles Adopted
November 1990

1. The NBNSC is intended to promote and recognize professional specialty practice to meet the increasing complex demands of health care through certification.

2. To achieve the above purpose, mechanisms must exist within the NBNSC for the recognition of specialty certification and the approval of their eligibility requirements and processes for certifying specialists.

3. For membership in the NBNSC, a certification board must demonstrate the existence of a relationship to a specialty organization or group that sets standards for specialty practice.

4. Uniform high standards must be achieved for specialty nursing certification. NBNSC-approved certification boards may fulfill this requirement by submitting upon application a plan that provides for:

   a. A specialty nursing practice certification requiring a minimum of a baccalaureate degree in nursing and a specified educational program in the area of practice to be implemented for *new* certificates by the year 2000.

   and/or

   b. An advanced specialty nursing practice certification requiring a graduate degree in nursing, or the appropriate equivalent, including content in the specified area of specialty practice.

(Courtesy of Hartshorn JC: *Nurs Outlook* 39:226–229, 1991.)

Conclusions.—The development of the American Board of Nursing Specialties as a means of setting national standards for nursing certification was examined. The evolution of this organization must be watched carefully to assess its effects on the consumer and the nursing profession. Certification of nurse specialists is the primary way of setting standards of care and ensuring their fulfillment.

Comments: The need for a National Board for Nursing Certification is questionable. Eight organizations did join together in 1990 to form the American Board of Nursing Specialties, representing occupational health, neuroscience, rehabilitation, nurse anesthetists, nephrology, and orthopaedic nurses along with the American Nurses Credentialing Center affiliated with the American Nurses Association. Six groups opposing the establishment of a national board for nursing certification represent emergency, postanesthesia, obstetric-gynecology-neonatal, neonatal-pediatrics, perioperative, and critical care nurses (1). These groups comprise a substantial number of nurses. The AACN had 4 points of disagreement with the national board: a need for the proposed structure had not been clearly established, the focus was on advancing nursing specialty practice rather than on enhancing consumer protection, there was no delineation between responsibilities of professional specialty associations and certifying organizations, and the requirement of baccalaureate education as a criterion for certification was questioned (2). The certification being discussed here is that related to *clinical practice* such as CCRN or CNRN, as opposed to *role* certification such as CNA.

The purpose of the CCRN Certification Program is to enhance the protection of critically ill patients by validating a registered nurses' qualifications and specialized body of knowledge and skills for practice as a critical care nurse. Currently there are 2 levels of registered nurses practicing at the bedside: one prepared at the associate degree (ADN) level and one at the baccalaureate (BSN) level. The AACN supports the BSN as the entry level into professional practice. Marlene Kramer describes future roles for nurses based on the typical and atypical patients' progress through DRG critical pathways (3). This system differentiates the nurse's role into the professional nurse case-manager who is BSN-prepared and the unit staff nurse who is ADN-prepared. A case manager would be responsible for planning, coordinating, and evaluating patient care as well as for managing those typical patients. Those patients following the typical pathway may not require managed care, but can be cared for well by the ADN-prepared nurses (3). This description of the role of the ADN nurses is ideal. The reality is that ADN nurses are delivering nursing care to typical and atypical patients. Certification was developed as a clinical credential to recognize those nurses who possessed requisite knowledge and skills in the area of specialty practice. If ADN nurses have the knowledge and skills and are providing the care, why should they be denied certification? Why is it even necessary to distinguish educational preparation as a criterion for clinical practice certification?—S.F. Wilson, RN, PhD

References

1. New Certification Group Sparks Vocal Opposition: AACN *News* November, 1:4, 1990.
2. AACN Certification Corporation Unable to Support Proposed National Certification Board: AACN *News*, February:1, 1991.
3. Kramer M: Nursing in the 90's: Trends to watch: *Nursing* 91, 20:67–74, 1991.

Subject Index

A

B

I

K

L

U

V

W

Author Index